CW00684142

An Atypical Journey

An Atypical Journey

V. Ronnie Laughlin

FRANKLIN GREEN
PUBLISHING
franklingreenpublishing.com

An Atypical Journey: Facing Breast Cancer Alone In The Middle East With God and My Tribe
By V. Ronnie Laughlin

Franklin Green Publishing
232 South St
Concord NH 03301
franklingreenpublishing.com

©2023 V. Ronnie Laughlin. All Rights Reserved.

All rights reserved. This book or any portion therefore may not be reproduced or used in any manner whatsoever without the express written permission of the publishers except for the use of brief quotations in a book review.

International Standard Book Numbers
Paperback: 9781936487547
Hardcover: 9781936487561

Editing: Heidi Jensen

Cover design: Heidi Jensen

Interior design: Kent Jensen | knail.com

Cover photo: istockphoto.com

Table of Contents

Dedication

An Atypical Journey is dedicated in memory of my parents, Essie and Hill, who taught me how to navigate life by just living their lives. I was privy to so many examples of patience, faith, discipline, perseverance, journaling, desire, dedication, determination, and the drive for internal motivation, all of which I called on during my cancer journey. I had both of them in the back of my mind every day during my journey. I also remembered my Daddy's valiant fight with lung cancer in the late 70s. He was a real trooper on his short journey. My Mom fought long and hard with breast and lung cancers as well. I know they were with me on my low-energy days, encouraging me just to put one foot in front of the other and keep moving forward—I did that! Thanks, Momma and Daddy; you gave me a beautiful blueprint for navigating life and my cancer journey.

I also want to dedicate this book in memory of my former Coach, Coach Kay Yow, who fought breast cancer with such vim and vigor, all while maintaining her Coaching position at North Carolina State University. Her very public journey with breast cancer set the stage for how to battle this disease and keep on moving and show gratitude. Even though Coach Yow lost her battle in 2009, ever since then, there has not been a day that goes by that I do not think of how she impacted my life. Having the opportunity to play for Coach Yow is inexplicable. She was a kind, caring, hardworking, meticulous coach who loved God and the game. Coach Yow taught me those skills through her examples. I channeled Coach Yow every day of my journey.

I always remembered her *Yow-isms*:

"I WILL, not I'll try."

"When life kicks you, let it kick you forward."

"Don't wallow in self-pity or you'll drown; you have to swish your feet and get out."

"Your attitude determines your altitude."

I made it my goal to keep moving forward each day. Before her death, Coach Yow had the foresight to set up a cancer foundation to advance the research for all cancers affecting women and to help those who may be underserved. To date, *The Kay Yow Cancer Fund* has raised millions of dollars for women's cancer research and education. Coach Yow was a crucial motivational force during my journey. I repeated several of her quips to keep me motivated and driven.

Also, in memory of my Mentor, Dr. Amelia Irby Hudson, I dedicate my book. Amelia taught me how to live life with no regrets. Amelia always had a positive outlook on life, even as she battled breast, colon, and pancreatic cancers later in life. Our conversations were often filled with philosophical quotes and life lessons from some of her favorite authors, such as Corrie Ten Boom or Khalil Gibran. Amelia was in my daily thoughts as I went on my journey. She had endured countless rounds of chemo and just kept moving forward. Before her death, our chats were a comparison of notes of treatment and procedures. Amelia had undergone breast cancer in the late 80s. There have been some amazing advances since her diagnosis. She always reassured me that I was getting excellent care and always made sure that I was grateful. I told her I would write a book to help others as a form of gratitude, and she seemed proud. Amelia taught me well. I am forever thankful for her taking me under her wing as a graduate student at LSU to show me how to live life and treat others as I wanted to be treated. Amelia truly was an example of a person living by the Golden Rule: "Do unto others as you would have them do unto you." It was Amelia who gave me some valuable "pearls of wisdom" that I summoned in my journey.

I kept my parents, Coach Yow, and Amelia in my daily thoughts as I waged my battle with early-stage Intraductal Carcinoma of my right breast in a Middle Eastern country during the COVID-19 Pandemic. I had to go to appointments and treatments alone for fear of infection from others. I could vividly hear them whisper little words of wisdom or encouragement: "Pace yourself but keep going." "You got this." "Look deeper to understand; remember—help others." These pearls of wisdom were part of my thoughts whenever I needed them. I am thankful.

Also, my book is dedicated to the many thousands of people who have battled cancer well before me. It was through their battles that research advances in cancer have been made over the years. They were shining examples of heroism and perseverance in their own personal battles waged before mine. They made valuable contributions to the research of breast cancer through their efforts. I am indebted to them and their sacrifices.

Lastly, *An Atypical Journey* is dedicated to you, the reader. If you are in the battle or about to go into the battle, it is my hope that during your journey, you will remember to stay in the moment and keep pushing forward. I pray that you may find your drive, dedication, determination and perseverance to overcome your battle through my words and examples. If you are a friend or caregiver, my hope for you is that you are the very best supporter and that you can understand the assignment and provide the love and support needed for your loved one during this time.

Foreword

I am not saying this because I am in need, for I have learned to be content, whatever the circumstances. I know what it is to be in need and what it is to have plenty. I have learned the secret of being content in any and every situation, whether well-fed or hungry, whether living in plenty or in want. I can do all this through Him who gives me strength.

Philippians 4:11-13 (NIV)

Get your highlighter, a pen, a notepad, and maybe your recording device. *An Atypical Journey* is a playbook on what to expect, how to prepare, and how to pray after the physician says, "Your breast biopsy is malignant—you have breast cancer."

I had the great privilege of coaching Ronnie from her freshman to her senior years of college. Hence, I know how she thinks, what she values, and what makes her tick. As you read her very personal account of her ordeal with breast cancer during the 2020 Pandemic while living and working in the Middle East, you will feel as if you are beside her, in her head and her body, as you read how she battled and experienced the disease, the medical tests, and the treatments.

Life-changing experiences often inspire autobiographies, but *An Atypical Journey* is not Ronnie's life story; it is her story about life with breast cancer. A beautiful and intelligent Southern woman, Ronnie was self-employed and living alone thousands of miles from home in a foreign country when her breast cancer diagnosis turned her life upside down. The cancer had inhabited her body. It threatened to take her independence, livelihood, mental and physical health, and maybe her life. True to her character, she became cancer's opponent with a "winner take all" mentality.

Every adult will experience cancer in some manner, whether personal, a family member, a neighbor, a colleague, or a friend. There is great fear of the unknown from when you suspect something is wrong until you hopefully hear, "You are cancer free!" The "unknown" is the combination of fear about your future health, the confusion from unfamiliar medical terms and practices, the stress of waiting for tests and test results, the uncertainty of the treatment's success, and the myriad of mind games that can cause depression and hopelessness.

An Atypical Journey is Ronnie's gift to us, a playbook or game plan on what to expect and how to prepare when someone you know begins the journey. Her careful notes illuminate the unknown, which eases anxiety and negates the many surprises. Her book contains personal insights, known as "Ronnie's Words of Wisdom," full of suggestions to help make going through breast cancer easier. Ronnie's lifestyle of regular exercise and healthy diet, faith, exemplary parents, influential mentors and friends, advanced education, and world-class medical professionals (and insurance!) were invaluable foundations. Regardless of where we are on the foundation spectrum, having a successful game plan will be fundamental. Ronnie's narrative can be a tremendous help.

To win against cancer or any imposing obstacle, competitors must engage physically, mentally, emotionally, and spiritually. Ronnie's game plan included action plans in all four realms. She researched online, communicated with close friends, drank gallons of water, ate high-protein foods, exercised, and talked with God. Philippians 4:11-13 became Ronnie's mantra—"...

Lord, may YOUR will be done." There is undeniable comfort in knowing that whatever happens to us is part of God's plan for us if we are following His will by putting Him first, giving Him the credit, claiming His faithfulness, thanking Him for all things because we trust that He will work everything according to His will (Romans 8:28). For Ronnie, a piece of God's plan is revealed in *An Atypical Journey*.

Enjoy getting to know Ronnie! Take notes—keep a journal—highlight the definitions—talk to God about it! Keep it close as a reference for you and your loved ones.

Thank you, Ronnie!

—Nora Lynn Finch
Women's Basketball Hall of Fame

Introduction

If you are a cancer patient, caregiver, friend of someone going through cancer or just someone who wants insights into what a cancer journey entails, welcome to my story. I am honored and want to thank you from the bottom of my heart for allowing me to share what I encountered and learned during my breast cancer journey in the midst of a global pandemic while living in a Middle Eastern country. In these pages, I'll share my process and my prayers and tell you about my people (My Tribe) all of which got me through the toughest battle of my life.

Before we get into my story, there are just a few things to keep in mind. This book is MY recollection of experiences over time as I navigated a cancer diagnosis during the 2019 COVID pandemic. Some names have been changed for the sake of privacy and some events have been compressed to the best of my knowledge; nonetheless, this is my story. Also, you may note that I have not followed the rules for the capitalization of titles. For my book, I have chosen to capitalize titles such as Momma, Daddy, Brother, Sister, Nurse, Doctor, Mentor, My Tribe, etc. as homage to the person and the title they bear. I felt that paying reverence to those titles via capitalization was appropriate. I am so grateful for each and every person, and for their impact on my life during this time.

Throughout the book, you will see sections called "Ronnie's Words of Wisdom." These are for you to highlight, make notes, ponder and gain inspiration. They are composed of advice, suggestions and "Ah Ha" moments I found to have a significant impact on me. Some of "Ronnie's Words of Wisdom" are tid bits of information I learned as I navigated the medical field. Some are just words of inspiration I felt you would need at various junctures in the battle. I hope they will lend a positive and uplifting perspective for you in your journey and support you through moments of doubt, fear and the unknown.

MY PROCESS

If you have been diagnosed with breast cancer, I want you to use this book to usher you through your cancer journey. The pages ahead of you share advice on what to expect, how to manage your treatments/appointments and how to stay strong. Get a pen and a highlighter and note anything in the book of importance to you. While these are my words, they are your pages to use as needed. I also suggest you purchase yourself a beautifully lined blank-page book to place your daily innermost thoughts, feelings and ideas in as you go through your journey. Write your thoughts daily in your journal.

I am telling you to do this now, because as I began to write this book, I would start a section and all of a sudden, the information I wanted to write was foggy. "Chemo Brain" is real, and I'll touch on that later. Sometimes, I could not recall a date or the order in which a procedure was done. I was relieved I poured so many words into my journals for later reference and you will be too.

I was thankful I captured my daily thoughts and ideas through writing, as my memories were often not as I had recalled. Information can easily be lost, twisted or even misrepresented in your mind when going through a traumatic event like a cancer diagnosis. The same can be said for the loved ones, caregivers, and supporters right alongside you who may remember things differently from how they actually occurred.

I actually thought and believed that I had "vivid" memories of what took place as I began to write this book. I am thanking God that I wrote down how I felt each day after the diagnosis, during chemotherapy, during radiation and after any procedure I had. My memory of the moments was a bit faded, but when I re-read my journal entries, I was able to go back to that event and recall the trueness of it. So, get your journal and start writing. You will thank me later.

Ronnie's Words of Wisdom

I had three journals. I did not plan it that way. I had always done a daily morning journal entry and one entry at night (two separate, beautiful, lined-blank books). When I got my diagnosis of cancer, I kept writing in my morning and evening journals, but I felt as if I needed one for the way I was feeling about my cancer diagnosis. My Cancer Journal was where I placed all of my feelings about how the cancer impacted my body, mind, and spirit.

I also had *My Appointment Notebook* that I have replicated for you as a companion to this book. I took mine to all my medical visits and suggest you do too. Living alone during a pandemic and battling breast cancer, I had a lot of time to think about the questions that I needed to ask the Physicians about my plan of care. I used *My Appointment Notebook* to keep track and you should too.

The accompanying *My Appointment Notebook* has an easy-to-follow format with one dated page with space for the discipline and Doctor's name at the top. There is a section for questions with space to write the responses. There is space to take notes during the appointments so that no information and details are lost. There is space for your vital sign information, next appointment date and next consultation needed. It is a comprehensive page with almost all the basic information that is needed to make sure good results are obtained at appointments. There is space for Nurses' names that provided the chemo and what side an injection was done on so that you could alternate the leg for the next appointment. For one of my meds, my thigh was the injection site. I alternated from left to right each visit to prevent damage to the area with repeated injections. There is space for the time the port was flushed, the dosage of the chemo drugs, the length of time of the chemotherapy sessions, etc.

My Appointment Notebook helped me to keep track of things that were important in my care. To this day, I take that same notebook to my appointments.

Ronnie's Words of Wisdom

I recorded voice memos for each of my appointments. At the beginning of the diagnosis period, the information was so vast and new, and sometimes I felt as if I could not keep up with what the Physicians were saying. So, while in the waiting room before I was called back for the actual appointment after my weigh-in and temp check, I would activate the voice memo to record the appointment. I cannot begin to convey to you how helpful this was, especially during my first visits with the breast surgeon and the new vernacular that she was sharing with me. I thanked God each visit that I was a Speech Language Pathologist (SLP) and had some medical terminology as a background that allowed me to chat coherently about my treatment plan. Later, I would get back home and listen to the appointment and augment my notes so I could possess a level of understanding and share the information with My Tribe. Maybe this "overkill" was the result of my profession and my dear Momma, who back in the day journaled and was a stickler for persevering, but it worked for me.

Regarding my work status during my cancer journey, I maintained my full caseload seeing children mostly online, as restrictions limited face to face sessions. That is, typically working five to seven hours daily. I did not cancel many sessions during my journey. Not one of my clients or their parents (to my knowledge) knew of my journey and still do not. I did not feel the need to tell them. Again, it would be so difficult to share my status, and to be honest, I did not want pity. I know that is a very pious thing to say, but I wanted to try and keep my high standards of performance at the same rate for my services provided and I did not want the parents to feel they were getting less because I was diagnosed with cancer. It was my choice—when you have to make choices—and you will have hard choices to make—for me, it was my right choice.

There were many days, as you will read about, where my energy was so low that it was all I could do to get from minute to minute.

Trust me, when I say low-energy, what I really mean is no energy, and by the grace of God, I was going from moment to moment. However, I kept moving. That is, I did my daily stretches, walks and workouts during my cancer journey. Some days, I moved slowly, but I did some type of movement every day. Maintaining my physical health was paramount since I was going to be responsible for getting myself to and from my appointments. It was imperative to me to keep moving and stay stretched out. I knew I had the mental tenacity for the battle. I also knew that I needed the physical stamina, as the chemo would deplete my physical strength. Again, I thanked God that I was able to keep moving forward mentally, physically and spiritually in my cancer journey. I persevered and stayed strong while plugging along and you can do the same.

MY PRAYER

After getting the diagnosis, I chose, first, to pray for the strength to be able to independently get to each appointment; that is, to drive myself to and from and still maintain my daily workload. As a private contractor SLP, if I did not work, there would be no pay. I had money saved, but that was not how I planned to spend my money. My prayer when I got diagnosed was this:

> "Heavenly Father, Son and Holy Spirit, thank you for this challenge that you have placed in my life; I am asking that you will grant me strength to drive to and from each appointment and treatment, and walk in and out of the hospital for my appointments and treatments and to continue to work each day to help others. I ask this in the name of the Holy Trinity. Amen."

My God is an awesome God, and I was able to drive myself to my appointments (radiation appointments were different—more on that later). I was able to work after I had my chemotherapy sessions. I scheduled the chemo sessions on Thursdays (in the Middle East, where I live, the work week is Sunday through Thursday). My premise was that on Thursday, I could get back home, have a light caseload, and have the weekend to recuperate. This worked out well for my chemo schedule. Even during the week after the chemo, if my schedule had a gap, I could catch a nap and regenerate for the subsequent sessions of the day. It was a plan that worked for me to manage all of this alone during a crazy global pandemic.

MY PEOPLE

At this point, I must share that I chose to tell only two very small subsets of friends. Some of you may ask why. My reasoning was this: I fully anticipated my stamina would be compromised during my cancer journey. I was basing this on how my family members and friends had fared during their own journeys with breast cancer. I saw various forms of their strength exhibited, and I observed that some days were worse than others; each day was a struggle for my friends and family members—and many had people to help. I surmised that if I was going at this "alone," kinda sorta, then I needed to have a small circle that I communicated with. If the list that I had to share information with was long, that in and of itself would be tiring for me. I had a group of friends that I named on WhatsApp "My Tribe." They were my closest friends and would keep my business in the group while providing support and encouragement. Providing updates during my journey proved to be daunting. So, I was relieved I had chosen just a small number of people to report to and give updates. I could communicate with them as a group, and it was one and done. My Tribe also knew me well enough to not hound me for updates if a day or two went by without any news. They gave me my space. Albeit hard, I would later learn that they all worried when I did not provide updates after each chemo session or the days following. But My Tribe "got me" and understood the assignment; often it felt like we communicated in a telepathic like way. They knew that I would reach out if I needed anything. I have to say that occasionally I did need someone to get me a few things from the supermarket on those low/no energy days and various members of the tribe would come through. My Tribe was absolutely amazing. My other subset of friends was near and dear as well and also got the update. Nonetheless, the subsets were small and manageable for me.

This cancer journey proved to be the most challenging thing I have ever conquered. It summoned all my strength, faith, belief, trust, love, insights and hope to win the battle. I found it was possible through faith and belief that God would not allow anything to be placed in my life that He and I could not handle together. As you follow my atypical journey with a breast cancer diagnosis in the Middle East during the 2020 Pandemic, you will see how prayer, positivity, perseverance and patience got me through.

Now that you know these pages are as much mine as they are yours, here's what you can expect.

This book is about my journey of being diagnosed with Intraductal Cancer or Malignant Neoplasm of the breast, stage II. The diagnosis was received in August during the COVID-19 pandemic in 2020. Receiving the news of breast cancer was difficult to say the least, but what was even more concerning was the fact I had no idea what my infection rate would be if I allowed people to help me with my appointments and health care. I needed to remain as healthy as possible. My immune system was going to be compromised and I needed to take precautions. I had to figure out how I (alone) would get to my appointments and treatments and stay healthy. Not only would this be a physical journey, but I also needed a mental component to stay strong. I focused my perspective to keep a keen mental sharpness and stay in the moment. I called on this perspective daily for strength to persevere. Maintaining this mental sharpness would feed my physicality and strengthen my mindset for the arduous journey ahead.

Here's my story ...

CHAPTER ONE

Children Learn What They Live

My Life Rehearsal

MY BATTLE WITH breast cancer took place in the Middle East during the COVID-19 pandemic. You may be scratching your head and wondering: "How did she get over to the Middle East in the first place?" "What made her go there?" or, "What was she thinking when she decided to work abroad?" Don't feel alone. My closest friends still wonder and cannot believe how long I have been here.

First, I would like you to understand what kind of person I am and how I became that person. Knowing this background information will have you nodding your head and saying aloud as you read, "Oh...I see now."

The title of this chapter holds the title of a poem my Mentor, Amelia Hudson, shared with me when I came to Louisiana for my graduate training in Speech Language Pathology. The poem is 'Children Learn What They Live.' You may be inclined to say, 'Children Live What They Learn,' which would take away the intended meaning from the poem. I know my parents did the very best they could with the means and resources they had when raising me. I know also that I learned from seeing and watching them be good people. I believe, no, I know, my upbringing and my experiences prepared me for my cancer journey.

MY DADDY

My parents were what I would describe as quite extraordinary. They lived and exhibited purposefulness in their lives. I was the third child born to my Momma (Essie) and Daddy (Hill); and the first girl. I always felt like my Daddy wanted a third son—ergo the name "Ronnie." I do not think I ever heard him call me by my given name, "Veronica."

Growing up there were a total of four children in my family, two older brothers (Vincent and Winfred), myself and a younger sister (Edwina). We lived in a modest home in the city of Greensboro, North Carolina. My Daddy worked at the P. Lorillard cigarette factory there, on the production line for twenty plus years. He enjoyed hunting, training hunting dogs, fishing, gardening and drinking *Ballantine* beer. He had lofty goals and aspirations to provide a good and solid life for his family. To do this, he took on a second job as the custodian at the United States Post Office in Greensboro. His schedule every day for years was, 8:00 a.m. to 4:00 p.m. at the cigarette factory;

home for dinner at 5:00 p.m.; off to the Post Office from 6:00 p.m. to 10:00 p.m. Our family had a schedule for everything. It was always adhered to, and we were always on time! These behaviors live in and of my being.

Memories of my Daddy are seared in my very soul, and for that I am forever thankful. Many people say I look just like him. I do not think as much, but boy, oh boy, do I have the headstrong personality and passion that he had for everything he did.

Growing up, I was his right-hand person when he worked on the car, tractor, and plumbing or when he was in the garden. My Daddy had a knack for figuring out how things worked—so he tinkered with things and usually fixed them. I enjoyed watching him problem solve and sometimes, I would come up with solutions right alongside him. Like when we were working on something, and I would see that he would need a wrench or pliers for the next maneuver. I would have them ready to hand to him for use. I took such pride in anticipating my Daddy's needs when we worked on things. He never said anything to me when I did that, but I smiled inside knowing I was right as he gripped the tool and continued to work. It was this development of internal motivation that would later sustain me in life.

My Daddy taught me many things in life, how to run a tiller, drive a tractor, and how to safely use a chainsaw, and more importantly, how to shoot a bolt action 410 rifle, a double barrel shotgun and a 16-gauge automatic shot gun—skills I boast about to others to this day. I was right beside him, as I gained a level of comfort for using, working and fixing things; not to mention the confidence it instilled in me when I accomplished things on my own.

Ronnie's Words of Wisdom

In your cancer journey, you will need to take pride in your small gains; whether it be eating when you may not feel like it, or trying to do more in a day than you did the previous day. Give yourself a "Way to go" high five and keep moving forward!

My Daddy enjoyed being outside in the sun, tending to his luscious garden and landscape. He found solace in the earth, seeds, water and sun. When it all came together and bore fruits such as watermelons, cantaloupes, pears, apples or vegetables like cucumber, onions, corn, squash, beans, peas or a beautiful landscape, he was a very content and proud man. I was happy too, knowing that I was a part of the planting, weeding and tending that was necessary to promote growth.

Ronnie's Words of Wisdom

Patience is key in your journey. There will be a protocol for your care that will be adhered to in the strictest of senses. Get your head around the fact that the journey is slow and steady, like growing a garden; eventually, you will see the fruits of your work—healed and feeling great!

As long as I can recall, we always had a garden and chickens, pheasants and quail. We used the chickens to eat and for eggs. There was nothing like Momma's pound cake made with fresh eggs. My Momma could prepare a really tender pheasant too and my Daddy used the quail to train his hunting dogs.

Even though we lived in the city, we had a garden. As a young girl, looking at row after row of beans, corn, okra or cucumbers to pick, I thought our garden was so large. To me, the young girl, the rows looked endless. When I returned home many years later and looked at the size of the land where the garden was—it was so very small. It's funny to realize my perspective as a child and my adult perspective are two very different beasts.

Ronnie's Words of Wisdom

This is why it's so important to journal. Your memory and perspectives will be affected by the chemo and your recall of information may not be accurate. You will have a different perspective when you complete the cancer journey, and the perspective may not be as it really was. JOURNAL!

Our garden gave us more than enough and my Daddy shared veggies with the neighbors, family and friends. He was very giving, especially when we had excess. He did not like to waste anything. He also sold some veggies to his fellow workers. Of course, my Sister and I picked the veggies, and weighed and bagged them for the sales. My Daddy gave us some of the money as an allowance. We learned to save and use our money wisely. We were young, disciplined entrepreneurs who were not allowed to spend our allowance on silly things; we had to save for things we needed, not necessarily wanted.

In the late sixties, my Daddy bought two and half acres of land for a large garden and a house and we moved to Sedalia, North Carolina. The family home is still located in Sedalia being tended to by my Sister after my Momma's death in 2019.

My Daddy had faith and patience that all the planting and landscaping he did would later grow and provide shade and even food (like grapes from the grape vines he planted) well after he was gone. His faith was deep, and he was right; the house is still in good shape with Edwina caring for it.

I recognized my Daddy's life as a simple one, yet full: Work, garden, train dogs, hunt, fish, go to church and relax with beer on the weekends. He was a good provider, generous and helpful to others and at times overly so. Often, my Momma had to rein him in when he got into the ultra-helping mode.

I saw my Daddy set a plan, gather what he needed, execute the plan and nurture it over and over again until his death in 1976. My Daddy gave me a sense of stick-to-itiveness and perseverance even during the hardest times. He gave me a strong faith base to believe in myself and whatever I set out to do; most importantly, to try my best in each endeavor. He taught me patience through gardening. As a gardener, you have to tend and nurture the plants and there's a lot of waiting. Can you imagine how hard it was as a kid waiting for a melon to ripen in the summer?

My Daddy was also a strict disciplinarian who expected things to be done in a certain way. If it wasn't to his liking, well... let's just say, I worked very hard to make sure it was, because I knew the consequences otherwise. I don't see his level of expectation as a negative thing. It prepared me to set high standards, set goals and instilled a mindset full of possibility.

During my cancer journey, I wanted the complete picture of

my illness so I could mentally prepare myself to be in the fight for the long haul. I wanted to know what to expect from the chemo, the effects of the drugs and radiation. My Daddy had instilled a mentality in me of a sense of expectations and preparedness.

My Daddy was just my Daddy. He did what he did—he provided for our needs. I saw him plan and execute his way to a solid lifestyle. Little did I know I would be planning and executing my life during my cancer journey using the skills I learned watching him live. It was the simple motto of "Children Learn What They Live"—I believe I did what I learned from my Daddy during my cancer trek.

I continually channeled Daddy during my cancer journey. When cancer related fatigue hit me like a Mack truck after round one of chemo, I thought about my Daddy and his drive, desire, dedication, faith and patience when times got difficult. He remained steady and took one step at a time in the right direction. I wanted to do the same.

After getting the diagnosis, I prayed to God and asked Him to allow me to walk in and out of the hospital for my appointments and treatments. It was my Daddy who was in my mind as I placed one foot in front of the other and slowly walked to the hospital through the parking lot to my many appointments and treatments. Desire, perseverance and determination were evident—I wanted and needed to beat this.

The qualities that my Daddy lived and showed me included: faith, desire, dedication and determination, sense of pride, generosity, helpfulness, perseverance and discipline. I am grateful to have seen those qualities in him during my childhood. Without knowing it, all my life I had been rehearsing for this cancer journey. I was armed with some good tools from my Daddy.

MY MOMMA

Now for my Momma—the kind and patient soul. She was a cosmetologist, or, back in the day, they were called beauticians. In the African American community, beauticians did a typical combination of hairstyling called the "wash, press and curl." This method was popular before relaxers and perms came into the culture for straightening our hair.

The family story goes—my Momma made a decision to go to beauty school after my oldest Brother was born. I didn't see her juggle Motherhood, school, and being a wife, but there were stories of her studying while holding my Brother, rocking or feeding him. She excelled in beauty school and got her license. My Daddy bought a house in Greensboro with an extra room and bathroom on the back just for her to have as *Laughlin's Beauty Shop*.

My Momma worked miracles in that beauty shop. I saw her exhibit patience, listening skills, organizational skills and guidance for her customers. How many times did a customer enter the beauty shop a little down or not feeling good about themselves or something in their life and leave in a happy mood with the fresh 'do my Momma had made for them? Too many times to count. Six days a week for many years she was a ray of positivity to her customers. It was my Momma's service to others that made her happy.

My Momma took pride in what she did and worked with the customer's hair until she had it the way she had envisioned it to be. She aimed for perfection day after day in that beauty shop. It was patience and perseverance that my Momma had as she worked with a young client squirming in the chair to not have that pressing comb make a burn on the neck, forehead or scalp of the child. It was confidence she exhibited in her craft, confirmed by the full appointment book. It was the personal pride my Momma took in always making sure she looked her best; hair neat and combed, and her uniform clean and crisp. Even when she was not working, my Momma was neatly dressed—perhaps that's why my Daddy nicknamed her "Neat."

My Momma took pride in everything she did. She taught herself to sew. One time, I saw her patience as she was trying to put in a zipper in a dress. It took her a few attempts, but she persevered and finally got it to her standard. She would always make a note of what she did so she could do it again. My Sister and I were growing fast; we were long and lanky. Finding clothes to fit us was difficult and expensive, so Momma solved the problem by sewing them for us. She later took sewing classes and learned to sew more complicated pieces. If there was a problem, Momma solved it; not to mention the money she saved.

She was a consummate problem solver. I once recall her making yeast rolls three times in a row, one batch after another, trying to get the texture, consistency and taste like she wanted. My Sister and I were the recipients of the baked batches that did not make the cut—they all tasted good to us!

Ronnie's Words of Wisdom

Problem solving of a different nature; throughout your journey, there will be a constant assessment and need for adjustment of your plan for better health. Be aware and involved in your plan of care. Using your intellectual hat will keep you on top of things in your journey. And remember to breathe; you will prevail!

My Momma flat out persevered in anything she did. When my family moved out of the city to the country she quickly learned to drive. She had the foresight to know that without access to public transportation she would be stranded. I must say, however, her driving skills were not that good, but she had given herself the independence she was seeking.

My Momma always kept a good weight for her height and watched what she ate. She was a good cook and used the fresh veggies and chicken from our little "farm" to feed us wholesome foods daily. We ate dinner together at the table every night. Again, being on a schedule was imperative in our household. It eliminated chaos and we knew what to expect. I have continued to live my life like this. During my cancer journey, I had many medications that I needed to take two to three days before chemo, and two to three days after. I made myself a schedule so I could check off the medication when I took it so as to not miss a dose—thanks Momma!

My Momma stressed the importance of drinking water every day and getting exercise. She practiced what she preached. She began each day with a nice big glass of water and kept that glass full all day. Little did I realize how important drinking water would be during my cancer journey to combat constipation. I love water and have always kept plenty around to stay hydrated, so I rehearsed this behavior too.

My Momma stayed active by working in the garden or tending to her flowers. She would haul buckets of water (weight bearing exercise) for the plants and flowers. Digging in the soil, bending and using her upper body strength were my Momma's core exercises. She kept moving. I thought about her often during my cancer journey when I pushed myself to keep my workout routine during chemo. I tried to walk each day, albeit slowly, but I kept moving.

Ronnie's Words of Wisdom

Hydration and movement are key during chemo.
The chemo drugs make elimination difficult. It is
important to hydrate and move/exercise and even
take some type of stool softeners to decrease the
constipation and pain.

One of the biggest impacts that my Momma had on me was her faith, encouragement and patience. We were Catholic. My Dad later converted when I was about twelve or thirteen years old. Every Sunday, my Daddy would drive us to our Lady of the Miraculous Medal Church in Greensboro for Sunday service. My Momma would have us looking neat and clean for Sunday mass. She always had her rosary—the one with the light blue crystals that she had until her death. She prayed the rosary every morning and night and before Mass on Sundays. She believed that everything would work out the way it was supposed to, and she never really got upset about how things turned out. She took life in stride. Like my Momma, I too would take my cancer diagnosis in stride and rise to the challenge.

Even in grief, my Momma was stoic and strong. When Winfred, my Brother, was murdered in Atlanta, Georgia in 1975, she got the news via a phone call early in the morning the day after he was killed. I remember talking with her when I got to be an adult and asking her what it was like to lose a child. She told me it was very difficult and sad for her. She said she had loved and enjoyed my Brother, her son, and his wild and crazy ways while he was here on this earth. Momma said his time looked like it had been cut short, but that was not the timeline God had planned for him. It was so comforting to see how she put my Brother's death in a place that made sense for her and kept moving forward. She encouraged herself to move on from the devastating loss. I recalled the conversation and remembered that during my cancer journey. I had to put my diagnosis in a place to deal with it and move forward; I was mimicking my Momma.

Ronnie's Words of Wisdom

You must move forward in your journey. No matter how slowly. Keep moving forward to better health and healing.

One of the most important things that I last learned from my Momma was to journal. She made little notes about what happened each day in the appointment books she kept for her customers. After her death in 2019, I was going through her things and found several of her old appointment books.

She had journaled or made short, little notes about when I went to college; she wrote down every time I called home and what we talked about. She had written quick notes to remind her what she did that day, what bills were due and how much she paid. I knew for sure I was going to journal during my cancer journey. It would be my homage to my Momma. This skill proved to be the reason I am able to write this very book.

My Momma's character skills included: faith, desire, dedication and determination, sense of pride, generosity, helpfulness, perseverance, patience and discipline—similar to my Daddy's. It is only now, as I write this book, that I see why they were a good team and how they really were compatible. They were similar, yet different enough to have the differences work in favor for them in raising four children.

When you grow up seeing examples of the characteristics/traits that I have mentioned, unknowingly the behaviors become imbedded in your psyche and are revealed as needed along your road of life. I needed all of them to make my cancer journey successful.

MY WANDERLUST

While I can claim the instilled characteristics of faith, desire, dedication and determination, sense of pride, generosity, helpfulness, perseverance and discipline from my parents—I can only hypothesize about where I got my sense of adventure that led me to going to the Middle East.

Neither of my parents traveled or talked about traveling. My Dad was an Army veteran, but I never heard him talk about travels he did with the military. My Mother liked to hear her customers talk about places they traveled to with their families, but she barely left North Carolina. There was one time we took a family trip to Virginia to an amusement park called Lakeside, and she also flew to the west coast for her one and only plane ride. A sense of adventure via traveling was not a trait I got from my parents.

In writing this book and trying to determine from whence my sense of adventure to take a leap of faith and work and live in the Middle East came, my best guess stems from going to college in the late 70's and hearing my classmates' talk of traveling.

As a student-athlete at Division I, North Carolina State University, playing basketball, I was enrolled in my major courses and decided I would continue with French as my foreign language. I had taken French in high school, done well and enjoyed it.

As the semesters progressed, I began to wonder and dream about traveling to France. I wanted to put my four semesters to the test. Looking at my meager finances, I planned instead to go to Montreal, Canada. That was my first trip out of the country— alone. This solo trip would prove to be life changing for me. It has always stood out in my memory and now I know why.

First of all, I was unaware that my bags had to be reclaimed and rechecked from the flight in Chicago. I did not do this and upon arrival in Montreal—no bags!

Secondly, I was twenty-one years old and did not know anyone, but I could speak French fairly well—and had nothing to wear or change into. I went to my hotel room, and I sat in front of the mirror and began to cry. I heard my parent's voices, my Momma's especially saying, "Ok... what are you gonna do? You gonna cry or find a mall or something to get a change of underwear and a top to wear while you wait for your luggage to arrive?" My Daddy was saying to me, "Remember this and learn from it so the next time it won't happen!"

I decided at that moment I could call on their strength to lead me and guide me through this fiasco of a trip so that I could enjoy my long awaited get away to practice my four semesters of French.

I went to the front desk of the hotel, and they were able to call the airlines to inform them where to bring the luggage. I then asked where the nearest mall was located. They directed me to right across the street. Off I went.

Keep in mind, this was the late 1970's and it was safe and common to speak with people you did not know—at least it was for me. I was able to purchase underwear and a sweater to tide me over until the bags arrived the next day. After my purchase I came across a nice couple and we began to chat about me being American, as they were Canadian. They ended up inviting me to a party somewhere within walking distance of the hotel that night. Being naïve and curious, I went and had a blast meeting some nice Canadian college students like me. My trip to Canada started out not too promising, but because I persevered and remained positive and patient it was life-changing! In the face of adversity, I persevered and found a way to have a great, life-changing trip.

During my Canadian experience I grew up and gained my sense of confidence, faith, adventure and curiosity. Since then, I have always enjoyed traveling, meeting people from other cultures, and learning things by asking questions to ease my curiosity.

Naturally, when the opportunity came to go to work abroad, I said, "Yes." I knew I could navigate a new country and make my way by relying on my sense of adventure, curiosity and social skills. All of my aforementioned parental influences and my natural wanderlust got me to the Middle East.

In 1998, when the offer came to go to the Middle East to train students in Speech Language Pathology, I looked to see where the Middle East was on the map. Once I saw it, I told myself, "That's a long way from home." I began to think about the adventure and challenge and signed the contract. I was going to be able to navigate in a foreign country, because I had learned through all of my life experiences how to be a decent human being to others and myself. I learned to lean into differences and try to understand the reason(s) behind the differences AND ask myself: Is the difference enough of a difference to make a difference?

As I faced battling my cancer during the pandemic, I was armed with many tools that would get me through the battle. I knew I had to persevere and to stay on top of things, as my life literally depended on it. But there was no one else to depend on, as the pandemic had isolated us all.

As I reflect, I see I was fully armed and prepared to take on the cancer challenge during the pandemic in the Middle East. Unbeknownst to me at the time, I had been rehearsing for this role all my life.

CHAPTER TWO

The Beginning

My Lumpy Breasts

FUN FACT, I have always had lumpy breasts. I can remember when I was twelve or thirteen years old, and my breasts began to develop. Surprisingly, I did not have real boobs until I was about fourteen years old. My Mother referred to this phenomenon as "late bloomer." When I did "bloom," it was more of a "bud."

During puberty, when my breasts began to develop, they were very, very, very slow in comparison to other girls my age. My friends had real cup bras. I wore a stretchy piece of fabric with straps. You could still see the print of it under my t-shirts—it was a bra, the rite of passage. I recall my little breasts (more like bumps) hurting as they developed, and I could feel a little knot in them when I felt them. I would later come to find out that the knot was called a fibroadenoma. Fibroadenomas can develop during puberty in girls or any age of women. They are little lumps that form in the breast and can be moved around. As a young pubescent girl, I was happy that I had "knots" in my breast. I thought it made my little bumps bigger.

FINDING THE LUMP

Fast forward to a sixty-two-year-old lady, single, living in the Middle East and a pandemic is happening all around me, finding a lump. Honestly, I cannot tell you how many months prior to actually going to the doctor that I felt the lump, but it was many months prior to the date I was diagnosed (August 23, 2020) that I found that lump in my right breast. When I felt it, I did not want to think anything except that the lump was a lump I always had. The lumps had been confirmed in several previous mammograms done in the states over the years. They had been labeled "dense fibrous tissue." So, I was not at all alarmed when I found this particular lump.

Now I know what you are saying and thinking: "Why didn't she go right then to get it checked?" That is a very fair question. I did not go right away because as I said, my breasts have always been considered to be composed of "dense, lumpy breast tissue." Any mammogram I had prior to the diagnosis resulted in "benign and non-suspicious tissue." There was never a need for worry or follow-up. So, when I felt the lump located at about the nine o'clock position on my right breast—I did not panic, but I have to admit, I had a very pronounced feeling in the pit of my stomach that said maybe this is something I needed to look at. Still, I did not immediately follow up. I allowed my alter ego, I call "Dr. Ronnie," to declare that we would watch the mass and check it when we felt like it and take it from there—do not judge me!

I followed the recommendations I gave myself; I watched and felt the lump—albeit I shied away from feeling it. My thought was if I do not feel it and feel how it is changing, it must not be for real. I promised myself I would "keep a watchful eye on it," which meant checking it whenever I felt like it and putting it into the nether regions of my mind in hopes it might just miraculously vanish. Yes, this was MY thought process—don't look at it, don't touch it, don't think about it, and it WILL go away, or at least be benign upon examination if I ever decided to go that route.

I was pretty successful at putting it out of my mind. I didn't look at my right breast when I got out of the shower or dressed in front of the mirror. It was part of my master plan for "eliminating" the lump.

I went on with life—working, socializing and maintaining a regular schedule. Of course, I did not share my findings with anyone—Lord forbid me from having to tell anyone. They'll wanna go get it looked at and that will open a proverbial "can of worms." I was not ready, nor did I want to do that. So, I kept my li'l secret hidden from myself and did not speak of it to anyone including My Tribe. Maybe they would find out if and when I did; or maybe they would not. I had not thought that far in advance.

NIPPLE CHANGES

My plan was working like clockwork. I had not closely looked at or checked the breast in months, as I recall, and I had not shared the info with anyone. One day, I caught a glimpse in the mirror. I was coming out of the shower, and I looked at my physique as I passed the long mirror in my bedroom. When I turned to get a full-frontal view, I noticed the symmetry in my breasts that I usually see, but I also saw my right breast areole was misshapen and being tugged at what looked like the nine o'clock position. My heart sank. Well, it did more than sank—it got full, and I did too, but I did not cry. "Aww shucks," I thought, "it's changing." Dense tissue masses do not change—or do they? A quick Google search (OMG, I googled everything!) revealed that I needed medical attention. A breast change such as the areole changing shape was an indication that something was NOT as it should be with my breast. I put on some clothes and fell on my knees beside my bed. I prayed that whatever was coming my way, I would be allowed the strength to survive and continue to help others.

Ronnie's Words of Wisdom

Googling for information can be a help and a hindrance. It is easy to find information that may not pertain to your particular malady. It can be misleading and cause some panic and anxiety. Information obtained can also prepare you for the jargon that will be given during your appointments. It can help with understanding the terms your medical team may use. When in doubt, just ask your Doctor.

But first, I needed to get my head around the fact that I just might have breast cancer during a pandemic in the Middle East.

I lay down across my bed, raised my right arm and I palpated the breast again, and it felt a bit different, maybe harder and a bit larger. With that realization of a change in the lump and my areole, I immediately knew I needed to seek not the opinion of bogus "Dr.

Ronnie" but get a real medical specialist to give me an exam, order a mammogram and go from there. I knew that changes of any kind in the breast are reason for further investigation.

Looking back on this cancer journey, it is very strange that I didn't recall the day, time or events surrounding when I first found the lump. You would think the day would live in infamy. You know, like a historical event where you remember exactly where you were and what you were doing when the event took place. I have no recollection of that day. Honestly, I did not want it to be remembered. Straight up—period! In my head for several days following the find, I was saying over and over, "I did not just find a lump in my breast." So, the next level of thinking for me was, "It's probably just dense tissue." I was going to continue to project positivity on the situation no matter what. Besides, all of the mammograms I had done in previous years always mentioned dense breast tissue. Maybe, it really was a piece of dense breast tissue? Yeah, that was what it was...right?

Seeing the lump change the shape of my areole prompted me to take steps to problem solve and get some answers and intervention if warranted. I had a Dr, Friend (Dr. Abraham, an Obstetrics and Gynecological physician) that I met through a friend here in the Middle East. I had his personal number and sent him a WhatsApp message—technology! My message was as follows:

August 3, 2020: "Hi. Dr. Abraham. This is Ronnie. I met you with Sage a while ago. You drove us to an event. Hope you are well. I was wondering if you are still holding appointments at XXX (local hospital)? I need a checkup. Kindly let me know if you are having appointments at the hospital. Many Thanks."

Dr. Abraham's response, which came about an hour later on the same day, was:

"Hi Ron. Ya, I'm there. You can call 012XXXXXXXX to book or book online through the website—see you soon."

And that's how it all got started.

I made an appointment with Dr. Abraham for a pelvic exam and a breast exam. The appointment was not too long after our text messages. On the day of the appointment, I can say that feeling in the pit of my stomach was ever present and I was praying for the best as I went into his office for my appointment.

The pelvic exam was unremarkable—thank God. The breast exam, not so. He palpated my left breast and those lumps that I had come to hear as typical for me rang true. "You've got dense breast tissue, and they are lumpy," he said as he completed palpating the left breast. I merely smiled and nodded as he held my breast. He moved to the right breast as I said, "I am concerned about this one; see how the areole is pulling/tugging to the right?" I nodded. He palpated the breast and repeated palpating the area at that 9:00 spot and said, "I don't like the way that feels. Let's get you an ultrasound and a mammogram to see what that is." He did not volunteer any more information. But reflecting on this whole ordeal, I wonder if he knew? I am going to ask him one of these days.

With this new discovery, I had to shift into survivor/beast mode. I needed to act intellectually NOT emotionally so I could follow the directions for the next step to finding out the status of the lump in my right breast. I put on my intellectual hat and proceeded to methodically navigate the hospital system in this Middle Eastern country. No more pretending the lump wasn't there. Now, a la my Momma, I shifted into problem solving mode.

CHAPTER THREE

The Ultrasound, Mammogram and Biopsy

WHERE I LIVED in the Middle East, you are required to get approval for any and all, and I do mean all, of the services that are requested by your physician. It is a process you get accustomed to, as nothing is done in a speedy manner. Navigating a health care system in a foreign country during a pandemic was challenging. My patience was always tested. The approval process involved going to the insurance office in the hospital or using the app on my phone, and submitting my paperwork detailing the services needed. A claims officer reviews this, and according to your insurance coverage level you can be granted approval. My insurance had good coverage. This was provided by my sponsor, which is the person or company that provides my accommodations (housing, transportation) and insurance in exchange for services provided. I still had to go through the approval for every procedure done during my journey. That got tedious, especially during the chemotherapy that was prescribed when you knew you were having X number of rounds, but you had to submit paperwork for each and every round. The process gave me an appreciation for the logic in the healthcare system in the United States and for good computer programs that were written to circumvent those types of problems.

Dr. Abraham had prescribed a breast ultrasound to determine if the mass he found was abnormal. He told me if the mass was deemed abnormal then a biopsy would be performed to take tissue samples for analysis. Dr. Abraham also prescribed a mammogram as another means of verification of the size and location of the mass that was in my right breast. I made those appointments for the next day.

The day of the appointment I was wondering what was in store with the procedures that I had scheduled for the day. I was going over all kinds of scenarios: getting a mastectomy, a double mastectomy, having a lumpectomy, getting chemo, going bald. The thoughts rushed in. I had to quiet my thinking before I entered the hospital, as I did not want my blood pressure to be high.

As I found my way to the Imaging Center at the hospital, my heart was racing and I was trying to look calm, cool and collected. I was praying, "God be with me, lead me and guide me, help me and may your will be done and allow me to be strong in this journey." I checked in and took a seat in the waiting room. Since this was during COVID, every other seat was open, and I chose a seat at an end so no one would sit to my right or left. My name was finally called, I went back and got undressed from the top only. I laid down on the bed with a hard sheet in that cold room. I didn't like cold rooms; my nipples were telling me loud and clear that the room was more than just cold. My mind began to race again, wondering a myriad of things: if my breasts would ever be symmetrical again, or if I would lose my right breast or lose this battle all together. I really had to get a grip on my thoughts and settle down and quell the negative thoughts. The technician, Hiba, introduced herself. She then squirted the warm gel on my left breast first. Thank God the gel was warm, or I would have hit the ceiling. I tried to relax, but I so wanted to see what she was seeing on her monitor (not that I had faintest idea about what the imaging revealed). Being the curious person I am, I would eventually ask Hiba why she kept going over the same place, zooming in and taking a photo, zooming in and taking a photo...over and over and over on my right breast.

Ronnie's Words of Wisdom

Curiosity can be an asset in your cancer journey; do not be afraid to ask questions and seek information. Be an advocate for yourself—this is your health/life journey. Own it!

FINDING FIBROADENOMAS

I turned to her and asked, "What are you seeing that you need to keep seeing again and again?" Hiba was a very beautiful Sudanese young lady and she looked at me as if I had asked her the strangest question. In all fairness, in the culture of the Middle East, most people do not ask questions, especially of professionals. But I, being the Westerner that I am, had a need to know what she was looking at that intrigued her and was perhaps...suspicious. Hiba was so nice, she said, "Turn around and look here," making the wand of the ultrasound machine turn at about 9:00 on my right breast, she lowered the ultrasound wand to about 8:30 and she said, "You see these impressions? They look nice and symmetrical. They are probably benign cysts." I could see what she was referring to and it looked like a lot of them were not quite symmetrical but more round than squiggly. The symmetrically shaped masses, I would come to learn, were called fibroadenomas (FA). They are typically benign (non-cancerous). They are caused by a deviation or change during normal development of breast tissue. I probably had these when my breasts were developing and lumpy long ago. The breast lobules become hyperplastic (over plastic). This change can be related to estrogen, progesterone, pregnancy and lactation. For my case, I would later learn they were related to my estrogen and progesterone. At menopause, they become atrophied (waste away); however, mine had not. The size of the FA is related to the estrogen level and that can vary. FA is usually found as a single breast mass during the early years of a women's life; thus, my dense breast tissue diagnosis when I was younger. On a magnetic resonance image (MRI), FA commonly shows as a round or oval shaped mass with a smooth margin and a demonstrated persistent enhancement with variation. On a mammography, an FA may also show as an obscure mass with equal density and oval shape, as mine did. They are solid, smooth and firm nodules. They can be easily moved under the skin and can grow up to two inches. They can get larger but at that point they may cause some pain. FA can be diagnosed early through clinical presentation and screening programs which will result in early detection of any malignant transformation and a good prognosis. In most cases, the FA does not require any treatment, especially if they are not causing pain, discomfort or anxiety. If removal is necessary, an excision biopsy (surgery) is done, and the mass is sent for analysis. At this point, nothing would be done with my FA in my left breast.

ONE OF THESE THINGS IS NOT LIKE THE OTHERS

Then Hiba moved the wand to 9:00 and said, "You see this impression? It's not so round. It has an irregular edge on it. That's what I am looking at and I am trying to capture a good impression for the Doctor to see. She will redo the procedure when she comes in." My eyes were locked on the asymmetrical blob that she had shown me. I asked Hiba if it was cancer and being the consummate technician, she replied, "I cannot say, I am only the technician. The Doctor will be able to tell you more." So professional!

Hiba continued to go over the site until she got an impression that she was pleased with, and with a few clicks on her keyboard, she had zoomed in and captured the suspicious looking mass on the ultrasound screen.

She told me to relax and that the images would be viewed by the Doctor, who would be in later for a closer look. I laid there wondering if the mass was cancer and what all the next steps would be. Right then, I decided to take a gratitude approach and be grateful for getting to the Doctor and having a knowledgeable technician speak with me, and for everything I had received up until this point. The Doctor entered the room after a swift knock to let us know she would come in. She immediately introduced herself to me as Dr. Noura and asked how I was doing. I replied, "Ok... so far."

Dr. Noura emitted a very positive and good vibe with an air of confidence about her; but not cocky. She was rocking some black patent four-inch Louboutin's and a nice print silk dress that was peeking out of the bottom and the top of her crisp white lab coat. I liked her style.

Dr. Noura said she wanted to repeat the ultrasound. She meticulously sanitized her hands and began on the left breast and then to the right. The left breast ultrasound was swift and efficient. On the right breast at that same spot, about 9:00 the repetition began again; just as the Hiba had done. Dr. Noura would place the wand and pick it up and go over and over the same area. She asked for me to look at the screen. I craned by neck to see the screen that was just over my right shoulder. The stylish Dr. Noura said, "this mass here, I do not like. It's not like the others—you see it is very irregular. I want to take a needle biopsy." She said she also wanted a mammogram as well. I said, "ok" and asked if she had time to do the biopsy now, as in today (the time was pretty close to the Imaging Center closing for the day) since I was already there. Dr. Noura was a bit shocked that I would ask to have the procedure done right then and there. She replied, "Yes, I have time, are you sure you want to do this now?" I said, "yes, I do not want to have to come back for the procedure and delay this any longer." I had taken the steps to get this "thing" checked and I wanted to begin to understand what it was and what I needed to do with it. In my head, I had procrastinated on this issue for Lord knows how many months. Now, with all indicators leading to a problem, I needed to address it, and as they say in the South, "put on my big girl panties" and do this. I know Dr. Noura was still in shock that I wanted to do the procedure right then and there as she asked me again if I was sure. Dr. Noura said she would write the order. I had to wait for the approval. I went back to the waiting area and waited for the approval. Approval came quickly and I returned to the exam room so that the biopsy could be performed. I was going to get closer to finding out what this suspicious mass was in my right breast that had caused my areole to pull away from the circumference of my breast.

Ronnie's Words of Wisdom

Honestly, I was moving fast with my thoughts, as I needed to have some information. I was operating in full intellectual mode. I was mentally ready to handle the outcome of a cancer diagnosis, as I was getting some answers as to what the mass was in my breast. I recall thinking, I have got to keep my head on straight through this—this is all on me. Try not to panic. You will find you are stronger than you ever thought you were.

Dr. Noura anesthetized the area of the breast, and the anesthetic was fast acting. I did not feel the pinch of the needle piercing my skin for the injection. Dr. Noura was smooth too! In about forty-five seconds—she jiggled my right breast and asked if I felt that, and I said no. In a matter of seconds, my right breast felt like a rock; I mean I could have taken a punch from the hardest boxer in boxing and would not have felt it. Reality was my breast felt like a rock, but it was not heavy; it was hard feeling but not a heavy hard feeling.

All that concerned me was I was not going to experience any pain.

Dr. Noura explained to me that she would be doing a core needle biopsy using the ultrasound as a guide to determine the site of the mass/lump. She also said that she would be utilizing a method called wire localization. She said she would be leaving a marker for the surgeon as a guide.

Dr. Noura said, "Ready?" I nodded. She inserted the core needle probe—a long, thin steel tube with cutting teeth on the end while Hiba used the wand to guide her to the actual site. She took a couple of samples—I did not feel anything. She kept the probe in my breast after taking the sample and ran a small thin tube into the probe. She told me this was a marker, to mark the spot for future reference. I would later learn that the marker would keep the spot indicated so that the mass could be measured, tracked, and observed after all of the treatment. She removed the core needle and the wire used to set the marker and placed a "plaster" on the spot. A plaster is what a Band-Aid is called on this side of the water.

Dr. Noura had placed the samples in a specimen jar and marked it with my identifying information. I asked to look at it and if I could take a picture—she agreed. It looked like white, spider/hydra-like, gelatinous masses with a bit of blood mixed in—that was probably a cancerous sample, I thought to myself. I was curious and asked, "Have you ever had a sample look like it was cancerous, and it not be?" She was stunned. She paused; with a look of concern on her face; kinda like, "how do I respond to this question." She took a deep breath and looked me in the eye and said, "No." At this point, I somewhat had my confirmation and diagnosis of breast cancer, but I had to wait for the results of the biopsy to be entered into the system. It would take a couple of days for the results to be read.

Having been exposed to a new vocabulary regarding my breast

tissue, I would soon learn the differences between a fibroadenoma and Intraductal carcinoma or the technical term—ductal carcinoma in situ (DCIS). This type of cancer occurs when abnormal cells are found in the lining of the breast duct. The abnormal cells have not spread outside the duct to the other tissues in the breast. DCIS is non-invasive or pre-invasive breast cancer. The cells that line the ducts have changed to cancer cells, but they have not spread through to the ducts and into nearby breast tissue. On the mammogram it shows as clusters of micro calcifications. These micro calcifications may show as white specks that are in clusters and have irregular shapes or sizes. This is what my ultrasound showed, as Dr. Noura so cleverly pointed out during the procedure.

Ronnie's Words of Wisdom

It is important to know the differences between the types of masses. Get a clear understanding from your Oncologist or Radiologist so that you know what to expect with regard to treatment. Do not be embarrassed or shy about asking for clarification of terms. I always did a bit of "Google research" before my appointments so that I could be prepared for the information they shared. When researching, keep a nice tablet nearby to jot down your notes/thoughts. It helps to go back and read through them after absorbing so much information during a doctor's visit or after a test. Not to mention, you will have better retention for what you read if you write it down and read it again. Having a frame of reference kept me more attentive and it allowed me time to process information. One of my favorite ways to ask questions was to use this phrase: "Can you help me understand..."—Doctors like this phrase, as it puts them into a comfortable teaching mode to help their patient gain a level of understanding in the care plan.

Dr. Noura told me to go to the mammogram room next door. She wanted to confirm the placement of the marker in conjunction with the site of the lesion.

Ronnie's Words of Wisdom

I was moving in slow motion as I made my way to the mammogram room. When Dr. Noura affirmed that she had never seen a sample look like cancer and it not be, I heard the wheels in my head come to a grinding halt and a whisper of "you probably have breast cancer." I had to keep my head on straight because there were things that I needed to get done. I needed to call on my Momma, "the consummate problem-solver" and my Daddy, "the rock steady" person who would plot out the next move. I took a second to digest what had just taken place. I relied on the strength and examples of my parents to help me navigate this new territory that I suddenly found myself engulfed in. I would need to draw on their strength, wisdom, patience and guidance for this journey.

THE MAMMOGRAM

The mammogram was the next step in putting pieces together to determine my diagnosis. In most cases, the mammogram is used for early detection or to identify characteristic masses or micro calcifications; however, in my case the procedure was being used in conjunction with the ultrasound to diagnosis a malignancy. The ultrasound had detected a mass and now the mammogram was going to confirm the location of the mass and that the marker was set in the correct position to mark the spot of the malignancy.

Because it had been several years, I cannot recall the last mammogram I had, I do recall I was in the states and I had been in the Middle East at this point for thirteen years, so, yeah, I was in need of a mammogram.

Now at this point, you might be asking, "Why did she not have regular check-ups and keep up with her health care?" I have no response to the question, other than, I felt fine and had not noted any changes in my breasts in years, so I felt there was no need to get a check-up.

Ronnie's Words of Wisdom

Behaviors like this happen, if this is you—don't beat up yourself about it. Taking it out on yourself will not do anyone any good. So, now, take your health seriously and get your annual check-ups. They could very well save your life.

The mammogram was simple. I am one of those strange people who just happen to love having my breasts squeezed by a mammogram machine—yep, weird! The tight squeezing of the breast does not bother me at all. Sometimes the technicians look at me strangely when I tell them that the plates can squeeze harder if needed. Do not judge me—I am built a bit different! I actually enjoy having my breast squeezed into a flat pancake because I have never had a bad or painful mammogram. I have several friends who dread the procedure. But, please have your annual mammogram done to detect any signs of changes such as calcifications, masses, or malignancies.

The mammogram is designed to give a visual representation of the breasts using various views to discern the structure/landscape of the breast and determine the tissue, density, identify masses and locate malignant and benign masses in the breast. Low-energy X-rays are used to examine the breast for diagnosis or screening or in my case, the location of a marker for future surgery.

Ronnie's Words of Wisdom

GET ANNUAL CHECK-UPS. Hindsight is 20-20 to say the least. My family history was indicating a need to do so, but I was feeling ok and felt no changes in my breasts over the years until I felt the lump months before I actually went to get it examined. I had always done breast self-exams and did not note any changes until the change in 2020 when I felt the lump, and in the months after when the lump began to tether my areole—the red flag was raised.

I am so thankful that my faith allowed me to call Dr. Abraham for the initial appointment and to get the proper treatment and begin my cancer journey under good care.

When I entered the mammogram room, it was very different from what I remember from years ago. The machine was smaller and more streamlined. The room was tiny, and the computer stand that the technician used was so compact and intricate. I had kept my gown on from the ultrasound procedure. I had to wash off all the gel solution that was used in the ultrasound, as it might obscure a good view of the breast tissue. The technician, Mia, who was Filipina, could barely reach the platform when it was raised to the height of my breast, as I am just shy of six feet tall (about 183 centimeters). On a good day Mia was about five feet, two inches. First, she marked my nipples with little tape markers that had a raised dot in the middle. I asked what they were for and she responded that they oriented the person viewing the results to the direction of the breast and the location of the nipple. The tape reminded me of the tape or suit that is used in CGI (computer generated images) as they kind of glowed in the dark. She then gently placed my breasts upon the small ledge and had me hold the handlebars of the machine to get the proper position for imaging. Then she closed the top part of the ledge down onto the bottom, asking along the way, was it ok? I reassured her that it was ok, as I felt no pain, just good pressure. Finally, Mia had my breast positioned properly and went to her control center wearing a lead like apron. She pressed a few buttons, and some beeps were emitted. She looked at the results on her monitor and said they were good, and the same procedure was repeated for the other breast. All this took maybe fifteen minutes.

To recap, at this point I have had the ultrasound, biopsy and the mammogram all in one visit. Now I needed to wait for the results. They said two days would be the wait time. In the meantime, I was thinking "I have breast cancer" and I went on the defensive. I Googled survival rate of breast cancer, watched videos of lumpectomies, mastectomies, and radiation. I was in full on intellectual mode—NOW—THIS CONCERNED ME AND I WAS NOT GOING TO BE CAUGHT OFF GUARD— AGAIN! I wanted to know all the answers.

Ronnie's Words of Wisdom

Gaining information about procedures, seeing videos of lumpectomies, or mastectomies will help you to orient to your procedures. I used the following sites consistently to search for information about my cancer, treatment, side effects, etc. The sites were the National Center for Biotechnology Information (ncbi) and National Library of Medicine—National Institutes of Health (nlm-nih). Together they provided a very comprehensive bank of information that was relatively easy to read and understand. It will give you the jargon to converse with your doctors and knowledge about your condition. It is empowering!

It was not until twenty days after my initial call to Dr. Abraham on 23 August 2020 that the lab reports confirmed the malignancy in my right breast. Intraductal carcinoma stage II. That is day that I want to forget but need to remember to be grateful for my life. Dr. Abraham called me to tell me the news. I could immediately hear it in his voice. But also, in his voice I heard a sense of hope and promise that he wanted to see me through this experience. The positive aspect of the diagnosis was that the cancer was caught in its early stages, and I would have a good rate of recovery and cure. After getting the news from Dr. Abraham, I went on the hospital app to read the details of biopsy. I got my news of having breast cancer not in a room at my doctor's office or with loved ones sitting around me, giving me comfort, no—it was myself and God sitting side by side. Remember, you are never alone on your cancer journey.

Dr. Abraham had taken the initiative and recommended a breast surgeon. Next, I had to schedule an appointment to meet the surgeon and discuss more about the tumor and the plan for excising the mass.

At the same time, what was in the recesses of my mind was Mrs. Alston (one of my Momma's customers who had a double mastectomy back in the early 70s), my best friend Cynt, my former Coach, Coach Kay Yow, my Mentor, Amelia my Momma and my Aunt Elsie—all victims of the dreaded disease of breast cancer. The commonality was they all had fought such valiant fights and had managed to maintain some type of semblance of the life they had led prior to cancer; I wanted that too.

Ronnie's Words of Wisdom

Breast cancer diagnosis during a pandemic; not a scenario I could have conjured up in my wildest dreams. This was going to take every bit of internal motivation, discipline and planning that I learned from my Daddy. It would also take my Momma's

> patience, perseverance and pride. At first glance, I felt overwhelmed, but when I had time to put on my intellectual hat, I knew that I had already lived and rehearsed the skills that I needed to get through this journey. I prayed and stayed focused.

The only problem was that I was in the middle of a global pandemic. All signs pointed to the fact that I was diagnosed with breast cancer just as the pandemic was starting to ramp up. It was still new, but even I was aware that I was limited in getting anyone to help me. Everyone was being ultra-cautious to avoid getting COVID-19. Yep, this battle was going to be with God at my side and communication with My Tribe. My daily prayer was for strength each day to get to the next. I had so many brave role models that I knew I had to fight and bear down and dare I say for lack of words... "Just do it." My daily prayers were that I be afforded strength to get through each day—it was not always easy, but I lived what I learned and went forth with all the tools I had to beat this.

CHAPTER FOUR

Meeting the Breast Surgeon

The Long Protocol, More Tests and the Tumor Board

IN THE DAYS leading up to the meeting with the breast surgeon, my alter ego "Dr. Ronnie" had already plotted the trajectory for my level of care solely based on Google searches and articles from medical websites like the *National Institute of Health*, *Mayo Clinic*, *WebMD*, *Medscape*, *Moffitt Cancer Center* and many others. I wanted to have the knowledge about my diagnosis and also to be able to fully understand what was about to happen to me over the next few months.

The information I gathered led me to think I needed a radical mastectomy and that I would have both breasts removed to ensure that the likelihood of another episode of breast cancer would not occur. Oh my! I know it sounds like overkill, but when you get a cancer diagnosis that significantly impacts your life, you start to take extreme measures to ensure you will live.

I did not have all the particulars figured out, but I knew what I would ask for when I met the breast surgeon. Based on my research I was adamantly opposed to a lumpectomy, as that procedure did not turn out well for my dear friend Cynt, who had died many years before. She had a lumpectomy performed and the cancer metastasized to her lungs then brain and she eventually died. I did not want that to be my fate. As Dr. Ronnie, I was prepared to fight tooth and nail for a double mastectomy; that is, based on my extensive research on Google. Little did I know I was thinking like a wacked out scared person.

Ronnie's Words of Wisdom

Use Google wisely. It can help you understand terms and procedures, but do NOT allow it to lead you to a "diagnosis" or "treatment plan." Be an informed reader/consumer and use the information as a guide to help you gain insights into your health and to have informed conversations with the doctors.

My head was spinning as I drove to the hospital to meet the breast surgeon. I went over the questions I wanted to ask and prepared to present my case by being sure to use the correct terms. I was focused, anxious and excited to start this journey. When I arrived at the hospital and parked, I took a deep breath and said a quick prayer for understanding, guidance, and strength through this ordeal.

I met my breast surgeon Dr. Rena, a very petite, young doctor for an evening appointment. It was so hard to see her face and know more about her, as she wore her mask, according to the COVID-19 protocols the hospital prescribed at the time.

Ronnie's Words of Wisdom

When I learned I would be seeing Dr. Rena, I "creeped" her profile on the hospital website for credentials. In the Middle East, medical training is a bit different than in the West. Medical students go to four years of undergraduate (UG) training, two years of internship training, two more years of fellowship training and then specialty training for two years. The students get some hands-on training earlier than Western education systems. Dr. Rena had done internships in the United Kingdom and the Middle East. I felt confident with her level of competence on paper. Understanding your doctor's background and training will help you to assess their competency level and give you comfort knowing you are in good hands.

I entered Dr. Rena's small, yet functional office located on the first floor of the hospital. Although focused and excited, I had done my research and knew what I was going to have done, but Dr. Rena's plan was not as I imagined. I was about to embark on brand new areas of knowledge, terms, and specifics related to breast cancer.

Dr. Rena allowed me/'Dr. Ronnie' to go on a rant and get all the nonsense out of my system. She listened and nodded attentively. At the end, she cordially said "ok, Ms. Veronica, this is what WE are going to do." Her voice had an inflection on the WE, to let me know all that I had said was nonsense and she would now present the facts and plan of care. It was during this exchange with Dr. Rena I bid farewell to 'Dr. Ronnie'—I knew I was out of my league on this one. 'Dr. Ronnie' would be retired, and the professionals would be allowed to do their jobs. I was in for an awakening.

Dr. Rena began by reviewing the results of my procedures including the biopsy, ultrasound (US) and the mammogram. First, she asked about when I noticed the lump. I responded that I noticed it changed about 2 months ago. I told her I had noticed the lump prior to that but my breasts were always lumpy, so I was not sure that what I was feeling was a lump or malignancy. Then Dr. Rena wanted to visually see my breast and palpate (feel). I took off my top and bra and lay on the table in the office. She palpated my breast and asked about the tethering of the nipple and areole. I told her I had noticed it in the last few months and that it was more noticeable when I remove my bra, as the bra tended to keep the breast intact. When I took my bra off, I noticed the tethering more.

Dr. Rena began to review in great detail the results of the ultrasound. She pulled up the image on her computer and zoomed in on the areas she was pointing out. She began by discerning the size of the tumor and the region that it was located. She explained, as The Radiologist had stated, an oval shape or regular shaped mass is considered to be typical; however, an irregularly shaped mass is a reason to explore more closely. She went on to say there was a thing called the "grey-zone;" which would be a cause for a biopsy. This meant the boarders of the tumor were causing concern and made it difficult to draw a conclusion about the mass. However, on my right breast in the 9:00 position, the tumor was close to the nipple. The distance was not easily seen and could not be measured so this led Dr. Rena to suggest an MRI would provide a more definitive picture, location and details that would all help determine the plan of treatment.

Dr. Rena was very thorough and after her questions about my family history, which included my Momma and Aunt who both had breast cancer. I asked if it was warranted that I get the BRCA (BReast CAncer gene) test to determine if I had the BRCA 1 or BRCA 2 gene. These genes cause an increased risk of various cancers (pancreatic, prostate and breast cancers) from generation to generation. Dr. Rena believed that was a good suggestion. She submitted an order for the specimen to be tested for BRCA 1 and BRCA 2. I wanted to know my risks of having triple negative breast cancer (BRCA 1)—a very aggressive and deadly form of breast cancer that would increase my risk of ovarian, pancreatic, gallbladder, bile duct and melanoma cancers versus BRCA 2.

Ronnie's Words of Wisdom

Your tissue sample can be used for various tests depending on your history. In my case, with my Momma and Aunt who both had breast cancer,

> further tests included the BRCA tests. Know your
> history and ask your doctor about all the tests
> that need to be performed to get a complete and
> accurate picture of your health status.

MOVING ALONG IN THE PROTOCOL—THE MRI AND CT SCAN WITH BONE SCINTIGRAPHY

I was just beginning my cancer journey and doing all the preliminary procedures needed in preparation for the treatment plan. There were so many tests that still needed to be done prior to any chemo or surgery. At times I felt as if things were progressing slowly. Just so you know, it's normal and it's all part of the process—it takes time.

Next step, I had to schedule an MRI (magnetic resonance imaging) and CT (computerized topography) scan with bone scintigraphy so they could look more closely at the tumor, determine the exact size and location, and determine if the cancer had spread to my bones. I learned the MRI would be with contrast. This meant a liquid contrast material would be injected into my vein via an IV (intravenous) inserted just prior to the procedure. This contrast would help highlight any abnormal areas of breast tissue or any other abnormal tissue. The ingredient in the contrast is called gadolinium. The contrast, once injected, would make a beeline to the cancer and show the exact location. I was instructed to drink plenty of water to flush the contrast from my system after the procedure.

The CT scan and bone scintigraphy (done with contrast) would allow the doctors to 'stage' the breast cancer—that is, they would be able to tell how big the cancer is and if it has spread to other areas of the body including my bones. This in turn, would help to determine the type and intensity of chemo treatment needed.

Ronnie's Words of Wisdom

The MRI and CT scan were important in helping the team get exact information about the tumor e.g., specific size, exact location and whether or not the cancer cells had metastasized (spread) to other areas. This information would be used along with the information from the tissue sample (protein composition of the tumor) in determining my chemo regime to ensure the best combination of drugs for my type of cancer. This hospital presented a well-organized cancer protocol that was thorough and logical, and it catered to my need for order and ability to follow the sequence.

I was able to go to the Imagining Center right after my meeting with Dr. Rena and schedule the MRI and the CT scan and bone scintigraphy. I had taken a picture of my work schedule, so I knew my free time. I would gauge and set my medical appointments around my work schedule, as I still had to have an income during this ordeal. Two days later, I had my MRI appointment. The CT scan and bone scintigraphy appointment was set for a few days after.

THE MRI AND WHAT TO EXPECT

Driving to this appointment, I was excited. There was no fear or apprehension, just the sheer thrill of going into the tunnel and hearing those sounds. I had never had an MRI, so per usual, I Googled what it was and what to expect. The information I read mentioned some people would experience claustrophobia and nausea. It stated that the noise could be unbearable, and some could not even complete the procedure because of the noise and/or nausea. With regard to the contrast, there was a small percentage of people who reported an allergic reaction, mostly itching; either during or after the procedure; my antennae where up for all of the possibilities. In my research, I wanted to find out if I needed to remove all my jewelry. Indeed, it was best I did. I have several holes in my ears and a dermal piercing on my chest that needed to be removed prior to the procedures. I did not want the magnetic field to pull out anything.

Before going into the procedure, I needed to sign a waiver stating I knew the risks and I did not have any metal objects in my body that may cause problems. I had to completely undress and slipped into a hospital gown. Luckily, the gowns at the hospital were the "good" kind; they were secure all the way around. An IV line was placed in my arm to prepare for the contrast injection. The MRI would first be done without the contrast and then repeated with contrast. The Nurse or technician putting in the IV line was good; he had a good "stick" as they say, and there was no bruising and pain in my arm. He taped the IV down and asked me to get up on the table for the procedure. I was under the impression that I would just lay on the table in the supine (head up) position. To my complete surprise, there was a little tray with two holes in it. Yep, my boobs would go into the holes as I lay face down on the table with my arms extended above my head holding onto to a handle. It was quite a surprise. I just smiled to myself, settled into a comfy position and the procedure began.

As the table slowly moved into the MRI tunnel, I was looking around; trying to see what the machine looked like—my curiosity was piqued. With the slow-moving table going into the tunnel, I began to have a hint of nausea because I was trying to see what the tunnel looked like. It felt like it began to spin. I closed my eyes and took a few deep breaths, then opened them again. Still a bit of spin was present. I decided I would close my eyes and try to sleep during the procedure. I nestled in and relaxed. Then the clanking and sounds began. They were a cacophony of what sounded like warning alarms at various volume levels, pitches and intensities. It was akin to someone banging on large pipes, someone knocking on a hollow door, all while in the background there was swishing sound. Somehow, I managed to drift off to sleep. I can sleep anywhere, even in an MRI tunnel. I was awakened when they moved the table out and called my name as they touched my shoulder. I think the staff were surprised I had fallen asleep. I really do not recall anything after about the first ten minutes or so of the procedure.

Next, I had to repeat the whole thing with contrast. The Nurse put the contrast into the IV and back into the MRI tunnel I went. The same clanging and banging and once again I fell asleep. It seemed like a short time, and they were moving me out of the tunnel. I got off the table and headed to the dressing room to change. I looked at my watch and it was an hour or so later than when I had entered. I just shook my head in disbelief and got dressed. I asked the staff when the results would appear in the hospital app. They responded in about two days. Since it was a Thursday, I could expect the results to be in the app on Tuesday, as the work week in the Middle East is Sunday through Thursday. I drove home, got something to eat and called it a day. In a few days, I would be back at the hospital for the CT scan.

Ronnie's Words of Wisdom

There were no discernible side effects from the MRI. It was recommended to drink plenty of water to wash out the contrast. I followed directions and felt fine afterwards. Start your hydration now, you will thank me later. Water will be key to your overall health during your chemo.

THE CT SCAN AND BONE SCINTIGRAPHY

A couple of days later, I would make the drive back to the hospital for the CT scan. The drive alone to the hospital was pensive. I talked to myself and wondered what this procedure would be like. I was not nervous but again excited as I had never had a CT scan. I arrived at the hospital and got checked in. I was called back to the scan area. The CT (computerized tomography) area was just down the hall in another section of the Imaging Center. CT scans are typically done to diagnose tumors, investigate internal bleeding, or check for internal injuries or damage. The scan combines a series of x-ray images from different angles around the body. Computer processing is used to create cross sectional images or slices of the tissue they are focusing on. The CT scan gives more detailed information than a plain X-ray. The CT scan is considered an asset to the cancer profession for its detailed imaging.

Dr. Rena ordered my CT scan (with contrast) to rule out metastasis of my cancer to my chest, abdomen, and pelvis. The bone scintigraphy would determine if the cancer had metastasized to my bones.

The CT scan was uneventful. I read that I could wear my clothes into the chamber, as long as there were not metal objects like snaps and zippers. I had worn the appropriate clothing so there was no need to change into a gown. It did not take long even with the insertion of the IV and contrast and was relatively noninvasive. It is similar to an MRI but quiet. The stipulation for the CT scan is you must remain still the whole time. Not hard for me to do, as I was certain to lull myself into sleep and just relax for the procedure.

I checked both procedures off my list and made an appointment with Dr. Rena to review the MRI and CT scan.

GETTING MY RESULTS

With all of these appointments I came to realize that I would be spending a great deal of time in my car. During those drives, my mind would race with "What if..." questions. For this visit, I chose to just let the information come to me and process it. I had grown weary of guessing, as that usually did no good.

My follow-up meeting with Dr. Rena was comfortable. She learned to appreciate my thoroughness (I always had *My Appointment Notebook* with questions, took notes and recorded the appointment), and I liked her use of Venn diagrams for explanations, as I was a visual learner. In Dr. Rena's office for the consult, she was very thorough going over the results of the MRI and CT scan and bone scintigraphy with visuals for me. I was thanking God for my Speech Language Pathology (SLP) background which gave me a level of understanding for the jargon she used; words like pre-/post-, names of organs, positions of perspectives (medial/lateral/dorsal), root words, MRI, CT scan, etc.

Results of the MRI revealed that the tumor was malignant; a second confirmation with the biopsy, as shown by the contrast going in a direct line to the breast area. Dr. Rena showed me the image. It was cool to see my bulbous breasts in a suspended state on her computer screen. Technology is amazing. Clearly, I could see what looked like a rope from the vein in my arm directly to the right breast at the nine o'clock position. There was no other direct line of the contrast going to other areas, as the cancer was showing that it was localized in my right breast only; no lymph nodes—many thanks to God! The lymph nodes would still be tested during my subsequent surgery—more on that later.

Dr. Rena continued with the results of the CT scan and bone scintigraphy. They revealed that my chest had no enlargement in the mediastinal area (the area of the chest that separates the lungs). This area is called the mediastinum. It is surrounded by the breastbone in front and the spine in the back with the lungs on each side. This area contains the heart, aorta, esophagus, thymus, trachea, lymph nodes and nerves. No malignant nodes were found in this area and that was a relief, as it meant the cancer was in situ (original place) in the right breast only. The lesion/tumor was 2.5 X 1.5 cm (conversion: .984 inches X .590 inches). That was less than an inch around. This measurement was different from the measurements obtained from the MRI. This could be due to the imaging itself. The bone scintigraphy revealed no metastasis of the cancer to my bones. The CT scan gives good spatial resolution (where structures start and stop) versus the MRI that gives better contrast resolution.

The clip/marker that Dr. Noura, the Radiologist, had placed during the biopsy was visible on the CT scan. If you recall, the clip/marker will help the surgeon more easily find the site on the surgery date. The tumor was described as being close to the skin and nipple. My heart, and lungs had no suspicious looking nodes; as did the abdomen with the liver, spleen, pancreas and kidneys

–what a blessing! The best part of the CT scan was finding out that my lymph nodes did not have any masses and that the cancer was not in my bones. This meant my treatment plan and chemo cocktail would focus on destroying the cancer cells in my breast.

Ronnie's Words of Wisdom

I would later learn that during the lumpectomy surgery the surgeon would quickly get a sample of my sentinel node in my right arm. It is located in the pit of the arm toward the inner part near the breast. I would come to understand that the sentinel node(s) are the first nodes draining a cancerous region. It (they) will be detected via a blue dye injection to determine if the cancer has spread beyond the breast. This is done during the lumpectomy surgery and the sample of the node is sent to the lab for immediate analysis while the patient is on the table. In the case of the node showing cancer, it and several others will be removed. If it is clear, nothing will be done. Warning: my urine was blue for about a day from the dye—no one told me this would happen—it was shocking and funny to me!

During my visit with Dr. Rena, she said she would order another test called IHC (immunohistochemistry) test to determine the type of protein receptors in my tumor. This information from the IHC test would help determine the medication regime post-surgery to combat reoccurrence of my cancer and cover all the bases.

THE ECHO TEST

The ECHO (echocardiogram) makes a graphic outline of the movement of my heart's valves and chambers through the use of a hand-held wand guided over my chest assessing my heart's anatomy and function. This would serve as a baseline measurement for the function of my heart. Some of the chemo drugs can have a negative effect on the heart. Having a baseline for comparison was a good move. I made the appointment for a few days after my CT and bone scintigraphy.

Again, my drive to the hospital was solemn and quiet. I wondered what the procedure would entail. All the tests I was having done were new to me, so I could only speculate what they would be like in reference to the information that I found through Google. I arrived to the hospital and reported to the ECHO area. I met the Sonographer. I undressed from the waist up. Once I had the gown on, and open in the front, the Sonographer hooked small adhesive pads with wires to my chest on the left side. These pads would register the timing of my heartbeat. After applying a warm gel, a hand-held wand was used to emit Doppler ultrasound waves to measure the size, appearance of my heart valves and thickness of my heart muscle. The hardest part of the ECHO was getting into the proper position so my heart could be scanned by the wand.

Once the Sonographer was set, he began moving the wand over the area of my heart. In the beginning, he had the sound on from the machine and I could hear my heart pumping with a swooshing sound. That was rather interesting. I asked the technician if my heart sounded ok. He nodded in an affirmative manner. The procedure lasted maybe forty-five minutes. It was easy, a bit messy with the gel (I had worn a cotton top that washed up easily in case gel remained on my skin after the procedure) and fascinating with all the sounds and images of my heart, its valves and chambers.

MORE TESTS RESULTS

The BRCA 1 and 2 tests took a while to return, I asked why they took so long, and I learned the samples were sent to the United Kingdom (UK) for analysis. This was my exercise in patience.

A few days later, I was able to access my file via the hospital app. When the BRCA results were in my file, I was unable to read the conclusion. I had to message Dr. Noura, my Radiologist who tried to see the results from her phone, but she also had difficulty. She said she would go to her office where she could access the report and information and later let me know the results. I heard back from Dr. Noura later in the day—**negative results** for BRCA 1 and 2. I was extremely relieved and knelt to say a quick prayer upon hearing the news.

Having a diagnosis of breast cancer is like doing a giant puzzle that did not have the picture on the box. I knew of the picture (breast cancer), but I kept getting new pieces to the puzzle, and I did not know how they would go together. I would have to wait until I got more pieces and then try to fit them together. What I would find is that some pieces could actually go in several different places—it is a perspective thing. The problem is my puzzle pieces looked different than everyone else's, and yours will too. The overall picture is that of breast cancer, but because of my genetic makeup, my puzzle would look different from the next person's puzzle and the next; my puzzle may have the same background or similar colors, but the pieces will vary accordingly.

Ronnie's Words of Wisdom

When I tell you I received an excellent level of care
during my cancer treatment in the Middle East, I
mean it. The hospital where I had my procedures
performed was state of the art. According to all
that I researched, the protocol that they were
following was more advanced than some in
the states. There are many good hospitals that
specialize in cancer treatment. Find out about ones
in your area.

After having results of the CT scan and bone scintigraphy,
MRI, BRCA tests, ECHO and IHC tests my case would be ready
to be presented to the Tumor Board. I was getting closer to finding
out what the plan of treatment would be for combating my breast
cancer.

THE TUMOR BOARD—WHAT IS IT?

With all my test results completed, my case was presented to the
Tumor Board at the facility where I would be treated. My breast
surgeon, Dr. Rena, gave me a quick tutorial about the Tumor
Board, what it was, how it works and its purpose.

The Tumor Board is a group of hospital professionals (consisting
of Pathologists, Surgeons, Medical and Radiation Oncologists,
Plastic Surgeons, Urologists, Gynecologists, Genetic counselor;
and anyone else specific for the type of cancer of the patient) in
various areas of Oncology and Medicine. They typically meet
weekly to discuss all cancer cases at the hospital and to determine

the best possible cancer treatment and care plan for an individual patient, based on the most current research and best evidence-based practices. The Board discusses each patient separately. The Tumor Board would have input from my Breast Surgeon and my Oncologist who would present my case and add a personal touch to the finite results that they were viewing. Things like the fact that I still worked out and was healthy were factors my doctors saw as positive prognostic indicators; meaning there would be a positive effect on my recovery.

My Breast Surgeon quickly and frequently reminded me that there was a protocol in place that would determine the best type of treatment for my specific cancer. Dr. Rena stressed that I would have to be patient, trust and believe that the Tumor Board would guide and direct my plan of care in the best possible way using their best practices.

Belief and patience became virtues in my journey. I had already asked God to be with me during this ordeal and NOW I had to trust in His will and the will of the Tumor Board.

Ronnie's Words of Wisdom

Tumor Boards are at all cancer hospitals. The idea of a group of specialists coming together to review and discuss your cancer case (and others) to provide the best multidisciplinary approach for your treatment plan with evidence-based information is comforting. Be sure to ask your Oncologist about his/her role in the Tumor Board's decision in your journey. Remember, this is all about YOU!

RESULTS OF THE TUMOR BOARD

A few days after my tests were completed, the Tumor Board met. I received a call from Dr. Rena. She said the Tumor Board had a plan for my cancer treatment. Dr. Rena was proactive and made an appointment with an Oncologist at the hospital as the next step in the protocol. The Oncologist would share the plan with me in detail and discuss the course of treatment. Dr. Rena said the treatment approach would be neoadjuvant therapy. This entailed me having chemo first and then another protocol for follow-up. The Oncologist would give me the details. The appointment for Oncology was in a few days... more waiting, but now it was waiting with much anticipation as to what this whole treatment process was going to be like. I was feeling a bit apprehensive getting closer to gaining insights into my treatment plan. The days could not have gone by any slower until I got to meet the Oncologist.

Ronnie's Words of Wisdom

My timeline began on August 20, 2020, with a visit to my OBGYN, Dr. Abraham. It is now September 28, 2020, when my plan is set by the Tumor Board for my chemotherapy rounds to begin on October 8, 2020. In less than two months (it seemed longer than that) my life was placed on a trajectory that I could not have imagined. Time will get distorted on your journey. Keep track of the dates of your procedures using your *Appointment Notebook*. It will be easier to access information when you have a hard copy of your appointments instead of relying on your memory. Your memory will get fuzzy during this time. Believe that you can do this, and you are halfway there!

CHAPTER FIVE

Meeting My Oncologist and His Team

J HAD TO WRAP my head around the fact that this journey was going to be extremely arduous and long. As I mentioned before, documenting it along the way saved my story and surprisingly I would refer back to my journals as a lot of information was not as I recalled. One thing was for sure; my faith in God sustained me through the entire journey. Many people say God does not give challenges to people that He feels cannot handle them. I certainly had not anticipated this journey, nor did I feel like God had chosen poorly. I truly believed and uttered the words "May your will be done" when I received the diagnosis. I did not cry, ask why, or get mad. There were some days (after round 2 of chemotherapy) going to my appointments that I had to park in a remote lot and measure each step I took very slowly. At point the cancer related fatigue had gripped my body; though my faith was forever in the forefront of my mind, body, spirit and soul. I BELIEVED I could manage this challenge during the pandemic alone, as the situation dictated. God and my faith did not let me down. WE made it through. I kept this prayer strong from my very first meeting with my Oncologist to my last.

I was grateful that Dr. Rena made my appointment with the Oncologist she felt would be a good fit for me. Once I had the name, I was able to access the Doctor's profile on the hospital website and see what his credentials were like. I had no reference to determine what criteria I would use to discern whether or not he was competent. I merely went on faith that I would be surrounded by a qualified, caring person during this journey.

The Oncology department was located on the top floor of the hospital in its own wing. It was adjacent to the Children's Cancer Department. When I arrived for my first visit, I had to pass by the Children's area. As I peered into the Children's waiting room, without staring, I saw such little bodies sitting on their parents' laps or in strollers. Their little lives had yet to fully begin, and they were given the challenge of battling cancer. I saw the parents look at their children with such love and promise that would allow them to stay strong for their children. I took that moment to say a quick prayer for them.

For all of my appointments in the Oncology department, I took the elevator that had me pass through the Children's area. I needed that reality check to keep me grounded and to know that although I had cancer, there were little bodies and lives not yet begun, who had to fight. This short walk past the Children's department kept me humble and most of all grateful. I gained strength to demonstrate the need to not relinquish to the horrible disease—not even with the added duress of enduring it through a pandemic.

That first day, I checked into the Oncology department and waited for my name to be called. My vitals would be taken, and I soon realized I needed to keep a check on those as well. The typical vitals are oxygen saturation, blood pressure, temperature, and weight. I got the results and placed those in *My Appointment Notebook.*

My name was called, and I was escorted to a room where a mask covered female Doctor greeted me. She did not say her name, but I asked her. Dr. Weeam, she responded. I soon learned that this pre-meeting with Dr. Weeam was actually an Intern who was practicing under the Head, Dr. Elyas, for training in Oncology. Dr. Weeam, as best as I could tell with her mask on was relatively young and married. She explained my diagnosis and probable treatment plan with precision.

Dr. Weeam discussed my immunohistochemistry results (IHC). My lesion/tumor was single. She further explained that I was HER 2 (human epidermal growth factor receptor) triple positive with my tumor. This means I was HER 2 (a protein) positive, ER (estrogen receptor) positive and PR (progesterone receptor) positive. The HER 2 protein promotes the growth of cancer cells. Dr. Weeam mentioned that my tumor was about 2.2 mm in size and that it was referred to as invasive Intraductal cancer grade 2. Grade refers to how the tumor looks (appearance); whether normal or abnormal. The stage of my tumor (stage II) refers to the size of the tumor and how it has spread from where it originated. My grade 2 cancer cells did not look like normal cells and were growing faster than normal cells. They were only in my breast—no metastasis.

The stage also takes into consideration what is known as TNM (tumor, nodes, and metastasis). This includes the size of the tumor and information retrieved from the sentinel nodes. Remember, the sentinel nodes are the first few lymph nodes that a tumor drains into located under the arm pit. At my surgery, I will be injected with a dye to trace the location of the sentinel node to determine if the cancer cells have spread to other areas of the body. If the nodes are found to have cancer cells, they will be removed. Dr. Weeam was quick to say that Dr. Elyas, my Oncologist, would go over the details with me. All indicators like the MRI with contrast and CT scans were showing that the cancer was NOT in my lymph nodes; however, a sentinel node test would be done at surgery for certainty.

Dr. Elyas entered the room. He was a tall, fit and lively physician. Once again it was difficult to discern his age because he wore a mask. His resume online would have put him in his mid to late 50s, but his physique placed him in his 40s. His arms were well defined, and his torso was trim. I figured, if he takes care of himself that well, he will take care of me too. To add to my comfort level and connectedness, he spoke very good English. Not sure what his nationality was, I did not care, as he had set me at ease when he entered the room and introduced himself and asked if we had met. Funnily, I too felt as if we had met before, but I could not call up the situation, place or time. Nonetheless, I was feeling like I was going to be in good hands.

Dr. Elyas was very personable and expressed his concern for my having cancer. He set me at ease by asking where I was from in the United States. We chatted about Florida. He commented on the good food in Florida, and I commented about the good Middle Eastern cuisine. He later shared that his two children who are doctors are practicing in the United States and doing well. He seemed grateful and proud that they were working abroad. Dr. Elyas was easy to talk with. A good bond had been established, as I would come to find out.

MY OPTIONS

Dr. Elyas was very systematic, precise and used thorough explanations as he reviewed my options. I knew he had given the same spiel on numerous occasions, but his delivery felt sincere and personal; as if he had chosen the narrative specifically for me. He began with my diagnosis—Intraductal carcinoma grade 2. He laid out my options based on the molecular profiling, from the IHC information and the bone scan from the CT. He proposed two options for me:

Adjuvant therapy—this was a primary type of treatment that involved surgery for the excision of the tumor, then radiation as prophylaxis (prevention), followed by repetition of the protocol of tests of MRI, mammogram and Ultrasound.

Neoadjuvant therapy—this is a type of chemotherapy approach that is used ahead of surgery to help shrink a cancerous tumor or even kill cancerous tissue that is not visible on imaging tests. When neoadjuvant therapy is used, doctors may also be looking at how the tumor responds to the drugs, and this can guide the treatment.

The Tumor Board had stated that the neoadjuvant therapy approach was best for my cancer diagnosis. This was good information to have and know. At this point in my journey, I just wanted the cancerous cells out of my body. If I had a chance of killing them first before removing the tumor, I was going to take those odds. The odds by the way, I would later learn were in the eighty percent range for survival for my type of cancer and my profile. Dr. Elyas was assuring and thorough and said on a couple of occasions during the meeting that if I needed some time to think this over, to take my time and let the team know which I decided on. Unbeknownst to him, I had already chosen to have the neoadjuvant procedure done. In my head, I was going home to

Google it, of course, to gain more understanding and insights into what it actually entailed.

Dr. Elyas discussed the delivery of the chemo drugs to my system. He stated I needed a port-a-catheter implanted in my body. This port would alleviate stress on my veins for the long hours that chemo takes for the many rounds. I needed to make an appointment and have the port inserted before the treatment plan could begin. My hope was that this would be one of the last steps before actually starting my chemotherapy. All I wanted was to immediately destroy the cancerous cells that had invaded my right breast. Patience and prayer would help me through the many steps to come.

In conclusion, Dr. Elyas informed me that I would have to schedule a meeting with the Cancer Counselor to review the various aspects of care, testing, the procedures, and diet as a patient diagnosed with cancer. Yet, another appointment to make.

Ronnie's Words of Wisdom

Your cancer journey will be directed by the protocol your doctors will use. The process is slow, methodical and well planned—it is specific for you based on the information they gathered through testing. You cannot rush the process; it does not go any faster than warranted. You cannot stress about the process; you need your mental acuity to stay focused on getting well. What you can do is focus on staying spiritually, mentally, physically, emotionally and psychologically strong, diligent and positive in this endeavor. It is not a sprint. It is your marathon for life, embrace it and pace yourself.

CHAPTER SIX

Cancer Counseling

Personal Care, Oral Hygiene
and Diet During Chemotherapy

BEFORE CHEMO

When I was diagnosed, I immediately went into to the hospital's chemotherapy protocol regime for treatment. This is standard per hospital policy. It includes a litany of appointments and prerequisites that were done prior to the actual chemo being initiated.

One of the prerequisites in the protocol was meeting with the Cancer Education Counselor, Mr. Ali. The purpose of this meeting was to get information about my cancer so I would get accustomed to what was coming in the form of tests, treatment, the vocabulary associated with cancer, timelines, procedures, dietary concerns, etc. I would also find out the order in which the treatment was going to be done. This counseling session shed light onto what to expect. I learned about what drugs were to be used, how the chemo would affect my body, how I may feel, what I would need to eat, supplements I should take and even how to combat constipation. It was an extensive and helpful educational lecture.

It helped me plan how I would manage my life and my body during the treatment sessions so I could have the most positive experience as possible.

Ronnie's Words of Wisdom

When you are in appointments, it is difficult to focus and take in all the information. I recorded every appointment I had, using the voice memo app on my phone. I knew with the chemo, there would be a high incidence of me missing information due to chemo brain, fatigue or lack of attention during the appointments. It's easy to do and you will be glad to have the recording after you get home and have time to process the information.

My counseling session with Mr. Ali would take place in the Oncology department in the hospital in a nice office-like setting away from the main area. It was secluded from the hustle and bustle of the patients coming and going for appointments. I was seated in a comfy chair in a dimly lit room.

MY SPECIAL COCKTAIL

Mr. Ali entered and sat down after introducing himself. He shared his information with me starting with discussing the common side effects of my specific chemotherapy cocktail. He shared how the drugs were given to combat my cancer and the importance of the anti-HER2 receptors destroying the cells.

The main drug—*Docetaxel*—was the "Mother" of all the chemo drugs in my cocktail and it could be responsible for any nausea, vomiting, low complete blood count (CBC), low platelets and overall decreased immunity. These symptoms would place me at risk for infections. This would be on top of the possibility of COVID. I absolutely did not want that on my radar in addition to the breast cancer.

Mr. Ali shared that I would be receiving some meds that were important to take at the designated times to alleviate nausea and vomiting. The medication was dexamethasone. I would receive a prescription for tablets to take two days before my scheduled chemo and two days after my chemo to quell my nausea and vomiting.

Mr. Ali shared some encouraging information regarding the number of people who experience vomiting and nausea while having chemo—It was a staggering 93% do NOT have those side effects. I wanted to be in that number.

Nowadays, in current chemo treatment protocols, there are drugs that are given before and after the chemo to combat nausea and vomiting. I am blessed to say I took dexamethasone and olanzapine for nausea and vomiting. I did not have any nausea or vomiting in all of my four rounds of chemo.

Mr. Ali also mentioned I would have to give myself an injection of filgrastim. This drug stimulated my bone marrow to make new white blood cells that are measured via the white blood count

(WBC). Having a good WBC would stave off a disorder called neutropenia (depleted WBC), a common side effect of chemo. He gave me instructions in how to administer the injection and said the drug came with instructions. That certainly would be something new and different for me.

Ronnie's Words of Wisdom

Your WBC will always be monitored before each chemo round. White blood cells detect and fight infections. Chemo can lower your count and place you at risk of infection. Getting an infection during chemo can alter your chemo round schedule and delay your treatment. All of my WBC counts were in the acceptable range during chemo. Be sure you know your WBC levels and if they are in the acceptable range. Giving myself the injection was not as daunting as I thought it would be. The needle for the injection was super fine and the instructions were clear and easy to follow—it helps that I do not have any problems with taking an injection. It was just strange to give myself an injection—but I did it and you will too, to keep yourself healthy and functional and your chemo on schedule.

MY DIET

Eating healthily during chemo is an absolute must. Mr. Ali's counseling session also included information on how to combat side effects from chemo by eating healthy foods; lower in carbs (one third of the meal should be carbs), with lowered salt levels as well as high protein. It was important to eat foods high in vitamins to provide energy for stamina.

I have always been a healthy eater, thanks to my Momma. I love veggies, nuts, fruits and cheese (I have a mild lactose intolerance). My diet before chemo was basically veggies with no red meat. I was still eating chicken, but sparingly. I had always considered going on a plant-based diet, but I was more of a pescatarian; that is, I ate fish. During chemo, I increased my intake of veggies, mostly raw. I ate salads (combos of romaine lettuce, kale, broccoli, cauliflower, cucumbers, onions, beets, zucchini, olives, avocados, chickpeas, black and red beans, aged cheese, etc.) with light salt and pepper and olive oil. I occasionally had fish to eat. My tastes for certain foods changed. During my chemo, I did not have a taste for tomatoes or almonds both of which I previously loved.

My go to snack became a nut combination of cashews (raw), peanuts, walnuts, pistachios, and macadamia that packed a good punch of protein. I ate natural ginger in my berry smoothies to boost my immunity. I have to say that I ate well during my chemo after my mouth problems got straightened out. Some days, I had mini meals throughout my day, other days I ate something for breakfast, lunch and dinner. My diet also provided the fiber content that would help with constipation. I still experienced problems with elimination despite my best efforts to maintain a high fiber diet.

My goal during chemo was to keep a healthy diet to avoid losing weight and strength. With focus and a plan, I was successful and did not lose or gain weight. My Tribe later told me that I never looked "sickly" or like I was going through chemo. They did say that I looked tired, which was the result of cancer related fatigue.

The importance of staying hydrated was drilled into my head by both Mr. Ali and my Oncologist, as hydration is key for keeping chronic constipation out of the equation. Little did I know, even with my valiant efforts to maintain my hydration and fiber intake not only would constipation be a problem for me, but it would be a big stumbling block in my management of my health during chemo.

Mr. Ali mentioned that it would be best to stay away from (for now) any raw, too hot or too cold foods as ingesting them could trigger nausea and vomiting.

Cancer Counseling is also where I learned about warning signs to look out for during chemo. It could be something as simple as checking my temperature. If my temperature got high that would be cause to go directly to the ER and let them know immediately that I am an Oncology patient. The high temp could be a sign of infection and that was something I did not want to happen. Mr. Ali mentioned common sense things like staying out of crowds. This was easy to do, as the country had been hit with COVID restrictions which limited travel and going out and around.

Ronnie's Words of Wisdom

As I pondered this idea of staying out of crowds, it was easy because it was during the COVID pandemic, but that also meant I would have to navigate this experience by myself, as I could not risk being exposed to people to who had been exposed to COVID. Having to go through this alone was difficult, but I called on the grace of God to lead me and guide along the way. You will learn that deep within you there is an intestinal fortitude that you will summon that will allow you to do things well beyond your preconceived notions regarding your ability. Keep staying positive and believe that you can move through this journey.

ORAL HYGIENE

During my cancer counseling, with Mr. Ali, we only vaguely discussed what happens with your oral hygiene (your lips, teeth, tongue, jaw, palate, and gums) during chemo. Luckily for me, I recalled friends and family who had difficulties with oral care during chemo. How could I forget the ulcerated mouths that made eating and drinking difficult and their complaints about food not having taste or losing an affinity for certain foods? I was praying I could be spared all of those problems with good oral hygiene.

When I researched oral hygiene during chemo not many sites mentioned problems with a sore mouth due to the use of fluoride toothpaste. There was information about oral soreness and sensitivity during chemotherapy. Suggestions included using a soft bristle brush, but few sites recommended changing the toothpaste for a non-fluoride one.

I was cognizant I had to continue my online speech therapy sessions thus, any oral hygiene problems I had would certainly be a red flag to my clients and parents. I did not to want to have to provide a reason for not being able to speak clearly or compromise our sessions.

When I did my first round of chemo on 8 October 2020, all was well with my mouth.

However, on day eight, post chemo, my cheeks felt as if had placed a large jaw breaker in them and sucked until my mouth was sore and had started to pucker. My lips looked fine on the vermillion boarder (the part where the lipstick goes) but on the dental side (close to the teeth) they were inflamed, red and tender. I was in pain on a level of about an eight out of ten.

I had to put food into my mouth with precision, so as to not hurt any of the painful parts. My tongue did not change color as many people reported had happened to them. It felt strange to eat and my taste buds seemed off. Thankfully, the roof of my mouth was unaffected. On top of this, my teeth shifted during all the rounds of chemo, and it warranted me to get my maxillary (top) retainer changed, as it no longer fit. Who knew that chemo could wreak havoc on your mouth?

Every day after day eight of chemo, the mere act of brushing my teeth hurt badly. I had gotten a soft bristle toothbrush, per the recommendation of Mr. Ali. As I brushed my teeth, it would just sting and burn to the point I wanted to eat ice chips to soothe the burning. It was not a burn like spicy foods, it was much more intense. It felt as if my mucosal membranes (areas in my mouth) were set on fire. Not brushing my teeth was not an option, as was not eating. While moving food around in my mouth was painful, the most intense pain always came when I brushed my teeth. The toothpaste burned and made my mouth sting. I tried adjusting the amount of paste I put on the brush, but nothing seemed to abate the pain and stinging. I needed a remedy.

I went to my community pharmacy and talked with the Head Pharmacist, Dr. Ibrahim. I told him I was receiving chemo and was experiencing oral/mucosal pain. I was desperate for help in any way. He was confident and sure in his response and labeled my problem as mucositis. With my background in SLP, I knew that meant there was an inflammation of the mucosal (mouth) tissue—yep! I had

THAT! He immediately began to inform me of the reason for the pain and discomfort when I brushed and explained that when you go through chemo it changes your body's chemistry and fluoride can become a culprit for a sore mouth. He recommended a non-fluoride toothpaste and oral rinse to clear up the mucositis.

I purchased the toothpaste and oral rinse he recommended—one tube of Eco dental non-fluoride toothpaste and Avalon-Avohex oral rinse. I was so nervous about using them; and yet hopeful I would not have pain. I drove home hurriedly and went straight to my bathroom to try out my new purchases that I prayed would be my holy grail. I squirted a small amount of toothpaste on my brush, said a little quick prayer and began brushing.

Oh my God... Oh my God... no pain. I mean NO PAIN! NO BURNING! NO DISCOMFORT!—out loud I thanked Dr. Ibrahim, my community Pharmacist! To me, He was a miracle worker. Who knew that fluoride was the bad guy in oral hygiene during chemotherapy? The rinse made my mouth feel revived.

My mouth began to heal, and my eating and drinking got back to baseline. It was probably about five days before my mouth completely healed. That was a big win for me!

Ronnie's Words of Wisdom

Oral hygiene will be a challenge during chemo. At the first signs of changes in your mouth, let your doctor know. Ask about using non-fluoride toothpaste and or an oral rinse to help with inflammation of the mouth—you can thank me later.

I used the non-fluoride toothpaste and rinse well after my four rounds of chemo were finished. I had read that your body begins to get back to itself about six months after chemo. After the six-month period, I cautiously used my regular toothpaste. It did not burn my mouth or sting and I have since continued to use my regular whitening toothpaste with no negative side effects.

To this day, each time I go into my community pharmacy, and Dr. Ibrahim is on duty, I always tell him that he was a true lifesaver for me. Along the way you will meet many angels and some in the least likely places, like a pharmacy.

CHAPTER SEVEN

My Direct Line to Chemo

The Port-a-Catheter

FEELING HOPEFUL AFTER meeting my Oncologist and Cancer Counselor, I was ready to move forward. All the steps were laid out—all I had to do was follow instructions, keep track of what I was supposed to do, take the meds I was given on the given days and times and keep my appointments. I loved the predictability of the protocol. It had order and I so love order. The next step was getting an appointment with the Dr. who would insert the port-a-catheter or port, for short.

The port is a device that was implanted in my chest wall, below my clavicle and above my breast (opposite the cancer site).

It is typically made of steel, plastic or titanium. One of the lines of the port of the catheter would be placed in my central vein called superior vena cava on my left side. The catheter intravenously administers the chemotherapy drugs for the treatment of the breast cancer and is used as a delivery method for the drug, as your veins are not equipped to handle the load (dosage—600mg or more) or the frequency (every three weeks; for a certain number of rounds of chemo) of the drugs. Upon entry into the vein, the drugs are diluted by the blood stream and distributed efficiently to the entire body.

The chemo drugs are specifically designed to kill fast-growing cancer cells. They actually change the DNA inside the cancer cells to keep them from growing and multiplying. The downside is that healthy cells are damaged along with the cancer cells as the drug(s) cannot distinguish the good from the bad. Each time chemo is given, it's a toss-up trying to find the balance between killing the cancer cells to control the disease and saving the normal cells. The positive outcome is that the normal cells tend to recover faster, and the cancer cells do not recover from the drug dose—this was the outcome I prayed for in my treatment. Attack the cancer cells!

I had a pre-consultation meeting with Dr. Deen who would insert the port. Dr. Deen was an older Middle Eastern physician. He said he liked my given name "Veronica." I think Dr. Deen had a hearing problem, but he had a Consultant (Intern) with him who asked the questions and took the information. Dr. Deen showed me the port-a-catheter device. It was much smaller than the ones I had seen in the video during my "Google research," and of what I recalled my Momma having with her breast cancer. My Momma's seemed to be bigger. I asked Dr. Deen if the size had been altered over the years, he responded with an emphatic "Yes, indeed, they are about a one third of the size they were years ago." This is a testimony to the advancement of technology in the field of cancer. It is ever evolving and changing.

Ronnie's Words of Wisdom

My Surgeon and Oncologist commented on how much they have to read daily to keep up with the most recent research findings regarding breast cancer. I felt encouraged, that information about breast cancer is ongoing and my team was keeping pace.

The meeting was quick. Dr. Deen told me that a small incision, about three centimeters, would be made here, as he pointed to my left clavicle/pectoral area. He would then insert the device into a subcutaneous (under the skin) pocket and connect it to the superior vena cava which would allow the chemo drugs to be administered. I asked Dr. Deen about the anesthesia. He said I could have general anesthesia if I wanted, but that the procedure was about thirty minutes and the recovery time from the anesthesia would be longer than the procedure if I chose general. Dr. Deen said the majority of patients received a local anesthesia at the site and a bit of a twilight anesthesia if needed. He told me I could do the local and the twilight and the recovery time would be faster. I chose the local and twilight.

After meeting with Dr. Deen, the insertion of the port-a-catheter was scheduled for 3 October 2020. This was a Saturday so that fit perfectly into my work schedule. I could have the procedure, come home and get rested and be ok for work later on the next day.

GETTING MY PORT

Of course, I revisited video of the procedure and saw that the maximum time with the prep before the actual procedure was thirty to forty-five minutes. In the videos, the sedation was more like twilight sedation, as the patients in the videos were somewhat alert. I figured, with God's grace, I would have the procedure, stay in recovery long enough to make sure I was stable to drive, drive myself back home, get some rest and be ready for work on the next day, Sunday.

The day for the insertion came. Remember the pandemic was happening and I did not have access to anyone I felt comfortable with driving me to and from the procedure. I was trying to stay safe in anticipation of my immune system getting compromised during the chemo.

In my notes on 3 October 2020, I wrote how I was a bit nervous driving to the hospital. It was early morning. I had alerted My Tribe (Angie, Angela, Ben and Jen) about the procedure and told them I would be checking in from time to time to update them. I wrote that I was nervous because I needed to be alert, aware and strong to drive myself back home. I quickly figured that I was in no hurry and when I got out of recovery, I could take my time until I felt steady enough to leave the hospital.

I arrived early in the morning at 7:00 am for the procedure and got checked in. As I was in the waiting room, I started to get worried, but then as I surveyed the people in the waiting area, I felt that my simple insertion was nothing in comparison to what these other people in the waiting area appeared to be in need of. One man had three family members with him. He was older and looked very tired and worn. Another gentleman looked relatively young, but his arm was large and flaccid and maybe he had a stroke or a burn. I prayed for a positive outcome for the people in the waiting room and for those who were to come that day. I merely asked God to be with me, the surgeon, and the staff and that His will be done. Little silent, quick prayers became a way to quell my swirling thoughts during my journey. Prayer centered me, as my focus shifted from the situation to a feeling of gratitude and reverence for the moment.

I was called back to get undressed and prepped for the port insertion. I had to undress. Yep, even my panties had to come off. Of course, I asked why. They gave me some webby undies that were not comfy. The reason for the webby undies, is that while under anesthesia, you may poop or pee your pants and if you have your undies on, they are ruined, and you may not have brought an extra pair. The webby undies felt weird, but I understood fully. I was grateful my gown was a nice one, good quality, and open in the front. It actually had a shoulder snap that allowed easy access to my left shoulder and chest area for the insertion of the port.

Dr. Deen and his assistant came in to chat and check on me. He marked the site on the left side of my chest just below the collar bone and quickly went over the procedure again. He asked if I was ready, and I replied I was. I said a quick Hail Mary and Our Father and was wheeled into the angiograph room. This room had interesting equipment and lots of screens that are used to view (angiogram) the blood vessels of the body. They did a sonogram (use of sound waves to see structures/organs) of my heart veins. The angiogram and sonogram would guide the placement of the catheter. I was injected with some lidocaine and my shoulder area quickly went numb. Then I was given a bit of anesthesia intravenously and that's all I recall, until I woke up and they were finishing the sutures and putting a bandage on the area. It felt like twenty minutes. Dr. Deen and his assistant said the procedure went well and all was good. I was wheeled back to the room that I had gotten undressed in and tried to relax.

The bandage was kinda large. I had a bulge just below my left clavicle area, but I felt no pain, as there was still some anesthesia in my body. I lay in the bed and got my phone and took a pic to send to My Tribe to let them know that all was well.

While I lay there, I shifted my focus to feeling well, safe, and good enough to get dressed and drive myself back home. The hospital provided a light lunch—a simple cheese sandwich with cucumbers, juice, water and a coke. I drank the coke, water, and the juice and sat up to see how I felt.

I decided to do a "Dr. Ronnie Fit Test" to determine if I was stable to drive myself back home. I stood up and bent over to see if I was dizzy—not dizzy—that was good. I tested my balance by standing on one leg then the other—did ok. I had to pee, and I walked, unaided, to the restroom—still all good. Sat on the toilet and did a few waist twists to loosen my back—still ok! Got up and tried to balance again—all good and walked back to the room. I started to get dressed and finished just as the assistant entered and wanted to know how I felt.

He was startled when he saw I was dressed and waiting to go home. He wanted to give me some Solpadeine for pain, but that drug in the Middle East causes me to have a nystagmus (rapid side to side uncontrolled eye movements) and to feel generally yucky. I asked if I could take Tylenol Extra Strength and he said that would be ok. I had that medicine at home.

I was discharged and made my way to the Oncology department to check about my next appointment, and they said I could make it online. I slowly walked out of the hospital, upon my own power and strength to the car and drove myself home to get some rest. On the drive home, I was saying prayers of thanks for the procedure and for feeling well enough to drive home. I was excited to see how this port would impact my activities and daily living.

GETTING TO KNOW MY PORT

Having the port in my chest wall was weird. It sat on my left side just under my left clavicle bone and felt wedged into the area that intersects with my shoulder socket. I knew it would take some time to get accustomed to a foreign body in my own body. I would have to revamp my workout routine to not put stress on that area until it was healed. I could shower and get it wet and after three days the bandage could be removed.

I did not feel pain until later in the evening. The pain was minimal and required no medication. I do not like to take pain meds and I was not in unbearable pain from the procedure, so no need for meds. I did not need extra drugs in my body!

The next day for my workout I did not do full straight-out push-ups but did the modified ones on my knees to make sure there was not a lot of pressure on my shoulder. I felt like I could not go as deep with my pushups, but I pressed until it just began to get tight and twinge. I noticed when I tried to extend my hands forward or up over my head that my range of motion was just a little bit limited, but I pressed on to the point of just feeling a twinge and stopped.

It took about three days before I did not even notice the port in my chest area. It was funny how quickly my body could accommodate to a change. I never had any soreness or redness around the site. I had to go back after about five days to Dr. Deen, who implanted the device, just for a checkup. He was very pleased with the way it looked and even gave me a "Mashallah"—This is an Arabic expression used when something good happens and you want to express a feeling of awe or delight. He was well pleased with his work, as was I.

Ronnie's Words of Wisdom

The port-a-catheter was not something I could have said no to. In my Googling about my cancer, most sources stated that a port-a-catheter was better than exposing your veins to the trauma of the chemo. My first round of chemo lasted over five hours—that would have been a big strain on my veins for that length of time. Get the port—it will make your life easier. I promise.

Next step, scheduling the chemotherapy that would course through the port-a-catheter into my system to destroy the cancer cells that had taken up a temporary residence in my right breast.

Ronnie's Words of Wisdom

The mental challenge of preparing to have chemo was a large part of the battle for me. My mental prep was going to be on several levels. Prayer was my first line of defense. I could accomplish anything with my prayers and faith. Secondly, my mental attitude was envisioning the cancer being destroyed by the drugs, giving me back my healthy body. Lastly, my Tribe would provide another level of mental strength with their words and messages of support, encouragement and prayers—I really believe that I was covered during my journey. Stay strong mentally; this leads to spiritual wellness which leads to physical wellness which leads to healing your body from the disease. Believe this—I certainly did!

CHAPTER EIGHT

Round One of Chemo

Getting Accustomed to the Protocol

I HAD TO MENTALLY prepare myself that drugs would be put into my body to kill the cancer. In my Google research and from the Cancer Counseling session, I knew there was a slim possibility of feeling sick and for hair loss. I also knew I had to take drugs prior to and after the rounds of chemo to combat nausea. By making a visual checklist for my schedule I knew would complete the assignment. Having done that, I was mentally armed for those things to happen. You know me by now and could probably guess I was not nervous, more like excited to see what the drugs would feel like going through my port and how my body would feel after each round of chemo.

In the car as I headed to the hospital for round one of chemo, my thoughts were focused on my body with chemo drugs in it.

Long ago, I had asked some of my friends who had chemo and they had told me that they had a "full" feeling; like a fluid filled body. I would soon be able to corroborate that or not. I was at peace during my drive and found these times alone to be the best to say some prayers of gratitude for the opportunity to get chemo to fight my cancer. I was also grateful for having the strength to fight the disease during the pandemic. I always resorted to gratitude when I could not think of anything else.

Arriving at the hospital and entering the place where I would get my chemo treatments was a bit different than what you might envision. Let me set the scene for you as to what an Oncology area in the Middle East looked like. It was very different from those in the United States.

The Oncology area was located in a wing on the first floor of the hospital. It was very quiet and serene. The staff consisted of five people, male and female from different backgrounds. There was a reception/check-in area where I got my room assignment for the session. Yep, there were private rooms; not the lounge chairs like in the states that are all set up in one large area. The rooms are very spacious and can accommodate a patient and about four family members comfortably. There is a hospital bed or recliner, nightstand, TV and two chairs and a large curtain that can be drawn to totally seclude the patient.

Privacy is very important in Middle Eastern culture. They take into consideration the whole family. Very rarely does a family member go to any appointment alone. Mother and/or Father, wife, husband, children or cousins usually accompany. The rooms can accommodate a family and I was happy to have a nice large private room all to myself, no family here for me during this journey; just positive thoughts sent from My Tribe. There was a total of sixteen rooms in the Oncology area. It was a very nice set up. One that I was always grateful for, as I mentioned my Sponsor, Hamza, (the person who employed me in the country) had given me the top-level insurance coverage.

When I entered the room for round one of the chemo, I knew the day was going to be long, so I blocked my clients from 9:00 am until 4:30 pm. The appointment was for 9:30 am and that would give me just enough time to get back home, rest if I needed to, and prep for the few sessions of speech therapy later in the day. I would keep those appointments in order to try to make my day "normal" or typical. It was imperative that I keep my schedule of work and not deviate from it, to avoid inconsistency of service for my clients.

Ronnie's Words of Wisdom

Expect to wait a while after you check in for your chemo appointment. The chemo drugs are made on an as needed basis. At the hospital where I was being seen, I would arrive at my designated time, but would have to wait hours for the drugs to arrive to dispense. My actual total time of getting chemo would be about four hours, but with the wait for the drugs the total time was six to seven hours. Be patient.

THE COOLING CAP

For round one, I had opted for the Cooling Cap which is used to prevent heavy loss of hair during chemo. I had paid out of pocket, as the cooling cap was not covered by my insurance. It was about $226, a small price to pay to keep my hair loss to a minimum. As

I entered the room, the cap machine was sitting to the left of the bed. It looked different from the YouTube videos I had seen, but it had most of the parts and components I was expecting. It did not have dry ice but was filled with cold water that was cooling to a low temperature.

With my wet hair, the nurse carefully put on one layer of the equipment that was connected to a medium sized hose; she secured that with my help and began with the second layer of the cap. This layer was made from material like neoprene, and it was heavy. It fit over the first layer and had a tube as well. The last layer was neoprene-like as well and was secured with a strap that went around my head a couple of times to keep it all in place. Once the Nurse checked the fit, she turned on the machine. It had a low groaning sound like an old window air conditioner. I could feel the water getting cold on my head. It never got so cold to make my hair have icicles like the videos showed, but my hair was cold and wet at the end of round one of chemo.

Once the cooling cap was situated, my first round of chemotherapy was about to get started. With your first round of chemo, they do the IV (intravenous) drip very slowly to start. I asked the nurse why the drip was so slow, and she replied that they have to make sure that I did not have any reaction. If the drip is fast, there may not be time to intervene; made perfect sense to me.

My chemo drugs in round one would be delivered through my port-a-catheter device. The Nurse asked if I wanted numbing cream to help ease the pain of the prick to access the port. I got the numbing cream and had to wait about fifteen to twenty minutes for it to take effect.

The nurse then placed a medium to large size surgically wrapped package on the tray table. This was a sterile bundle that would be unwrapped and used for my chemo. She began to unwrap the package. The first thing she took out was tongs to unwrap the layers so as to not touch any of the sterile items. She took out a heavy paper gown and large rubber gloves and donned those. On the next layer of the unwrapping were the cleaning materials to clean my port site. She used another set of tongs to remove those and place them in the sterile field. Betadine solution on a gauze pad was used to wipe my port site clean. Betadine is the hospital standard antiseptic solution. It is used to prepare skin for surgery. It also reduces bacteria on the skin to prevent infection. The active ingredient is povidone-iodine. It is active against many pathogens (germs). Be prepared, this is a rich, dark brown, shiny, viscous liquid that has no odor. It was then wiped dry.

Next the Nurse accessed my port. The area around the port was numb from the cream. I was asked to take a deep breath and she punctured the silicone bubble or septum of the port for access with a firm press into the port. I felt the pressure of the pushing of the needle, but no pain—the numbing cream worked!

With the port accessed, she then flushed it with saline which prepped the line for the chemo drugs. The first bag of my chemo drug, docetaxel, was hanging on the IV pole beside the bed. It would soon be connected and begin the slow drip. Also on the drip stand, or IV pole, was a bag of saline and diphenhydramine to help quell the nausea. The Nurse asked if I had taken my dexamethasone two days before my chemo. I told her that I had, and I would take it two days after my chemo to make sure I did not experience nausea or vomiting.

My docetaxel had the job of running interference with the growth of cancer cells. The downside of that drug is it does not discriminate how it affects cells; it targets healthy and cancerous cells. I just wanted it to help me have a healthy body again.

The nurse asked if I was ready for the first bag of the chemotherapy drug. I said I was and honestly, I was kind of excited to see what the procedure would look like.

The drip was very slow, and it appeared I was not having a reaction, no swelling, fever or itching. When my vitals were taken, they revealed I was doing well. After about thirty minutes, the nurse increased the drip and soon (about an hour and a half) the first bag was finished. The bag of docetaxel was disposed of properly and carefully in a special container.

Suddenly, it dawned on me I had a chemotherapy drug coursing through my body, attacking the cancer cells in my right breast to kill them and make me healthy again. I prayed that the drugs were fighting valiantly.

Ronnie's Words of Wisdom

So this was chemotherapy. As I sat alone in my hospital room, I was getting chemo during a pandemic in a Middle Eastern country. I was not sad; I was grateful and felt blessed that I had the opportunity to get the care I needed. After that first bag was finished, I said a prayer of thanks for making it to this point. I knew I had a long road ahead of me, but I was in the moment and dealing with the now, just as my Daddy or Momma would have done with any life situation they faced; be grateful and learn, it would surely happen again.

One drug down; on to the next bag—pertuzumab. My port line was flushed again with saline, and the second bag was started, ever so slowly.

My pertuzumab was going to work by locking onto the HER2 (human epidermal growth factor receptor 2) receptors on my cancer cells in the tumor by killing/blocking them thus stopping them from growing. I had HER2 triple positive cancer which meant my tumor had estrogen and progesterone receptors, as well as too many HER2 receptors. In essence, my body was making food in the form of a protein for the cancer to live on. I needed a drug that would kill the receptors to stop the growth of the cancer.

The drip was very slow, and the nurse waited about thirty minutes again to ensure there was no reaction. My vitals were taken and once again revealed I was handling it well. Later, she entered the room and checked that I was doing ok, with no signs or symptoms of a reaction. At that point the drip was increased. In about an hour and a half, the second bag was completed and disposed of properly.

It had taken roughly three hours for all the chemo drugs to drip into my body. But I was far from being done for my first round of chemotherapy.

All the intravenous lines were stopped. My port was flushed out and heparin was injected to keep the line patent (open) so it would not clog between now and the next round.

Ronnie's Words of Wisdom

A port should be flushed every four to six weeks if it is not being accessed. If it is not flushed, there is a chance of infection.

The nurse assured me that the next rounds would be faster. I was trying to calculate the time it took, so I could plan my work schedule. I knew I would need time to come home and rest before beginning my day of seeing my clients.

Being a planner, I scheduled all of my chemo rounds to be on Thursdays. This would give me the weekend to recoup and figure out how I was feeling before I had to face another week of work. It made sense to me.

Ronnie's Words of Wisdom

I had to figure out a way to work and have my chemotherapy. Having the responsibility of providing speech therapy to several children and families gave me focus. This kept me busy. Having to work and schedule the chemo sessions really helped to keep my mind occupied and not focus on me. I had to shift my mindset to focus on my clients. I needed to be cognizant of helping them make progress and stay positive and upbeat during the sessions. In hindsight, having work that had to be done was a Godsend for me.

My first round of chemo was not quite over yet. Next up was an injection that was known as a "hot shot." That means that the medication goes into your body and can feel hot as it enters if it is injected too fast. To prevent this, the nurse is required to administer the injection very, very, very slowly. This drug was called trastuzumab aka Herceptin. This drug is known as a targeted therapy drug. It changes the way cells work and helps to stop cancer from growing and spreading. My trastuzumab had the assignment of helping to control the cancer cells that contain high amounts of HER2. I had a high level of HER2 positive receptors with my cancer.

I had worn loose pants so I could just pull up my pant leg for the injection in my thigh (I had to alternate sides with each injection so as to not cause trauma to the area)—I kept track of that in *My Appointment Notebook*. Because the injection may be painful, the nurse asked me if I wanted the numbing cream. I had her apply the cream and waited for the numbing to take effect

Ronnie's Words of Wisdom

I toyed with the idea of not getting the numbing cream to determine what kind of pain there was with the injection and the piercing of my port. It was not until later in round three that I stopped the numbing cream for both procedures. For me, the pain was not intense without the cream. I have a high tolerance for pain. Always do what you feel is best for your comfort level

When the nurse returned, she sat on the side of the bed with me. She gloved up and gave me instructions on when to tell her to stop if I felt any burning or pain. I was ready.

She cleaned the area and started the injection. It was soooo slow, but I was not complaining. I did not want to experience any pain or feel the heat that the injection could create. After every maybe ten seconds she asked if I felt any discomfort—I did not.

She continued with the injection for almost six minutes—that is a very slow injection. I know this exact time because I videotaped it. She did well, as I felt no pain or discomfort during the ordeal.

Ronnie's Words of Wisdom

I was always wondering about procedures. I had the nurse push the injection in one of my later rounds just a bit—Wowie! It was hot. It felt like a hot pin had been stuck on my thigh. I signaled for the nurse to stop. We both giggled. I allowed her to continue with the slow injection rate.

I was still not done and could not claim and celebrate completion of my first round of chemo. I had to remove the cooling cap equipment before I could be dismissed. The Nurses removed all the equipment. Total time in the Chemo area: approximately seven hours (with the wait for the drugs from pharmacy).

I was praying that my hair loss would be minimal so that I could avoid having to explain my hair loss to anyone. I was not very optimistic that the cooling cap was going to be effective. I dried and slicked back my hair as well as I could and wrapped it in a head scarf so no one would know that I just had a round of chemo.

I felt tired but I think it was from the anticipation of the procedure. I was thanking God that I felt ok after round one and was able to drive home. I had enough energy to drive myself to get groceries. I felt ok in the moments right after round one of chemo. A little tired, but not exhausted. I could get home, get some rest before my afternoon sessions began.

Now, I have to insert here that I walked and moved slowly through the supermarket; more slowly than what I was typically accustomed to. I am almost six feet tall with an inseam of thirty-six inches; my stride is L-O-N-G! Right after round one, as I walked through the supermarket to pick up a few things, my stride was deliberate and paced. I knew I could not rush through and walk fast, as I might deplete my energy. I wanted to measure my steps, one at a time, and to walk more slowly, cautiously; actually, taking in the elements of the environment—something I typically had not been doing. My gait did not appear to be "sickly," or that I was in pain or hurting; it was just a nice stride to conserve my energy. So far, I felt ok, and that was good for me—just having chemotherapy drugs pumped into my body.

Ronnie's Words of Wisdom

The first round of chemo is a major step in your cancer journey. Be sure to give yourself credit for this amazing accomplishment. You are mightier than you think you are. Chemo is not for the faint of heart. You did this! Onward to the next round with the same positivity and vigor!

Getting home, I was tired, but a quick nap had me feeling less tired. I was glad it was the end of my work week. My sessions went well, and I was able to say that I drove myself to and from my chemo session and kept my work schedule—I was proud of myself. This would not be the last moment of pride that I would feel on this journey.

Ronnie's Words of Wisdom

Cancer Related Fatigue (CRF) as I would later learn it was called, set in on day two post-chemo round one and did not subside until day ten. My oral hygiene began to breakdown on day eight post chemo of round one. Lastly, I had an allergic reaction (severe itching on my upper torso; front and back and neck) on day ten post chemo round one to one of the chemo drugs. That was a battle within a battle, as my Oncologist and I had to determine what drug was causing the itching and was it one that could be eliminated and still achieve the response of killing the cancer cells. The war had been waged.

BEYOND TIRED—MEET *THE BEAST*

According to any site that you Google, Cancer related fatigue (CRF) is a condition which is known as a common side effect of chemotherapy and its treatment. CRF is a fatigue that is more severe, more persistent and more debilitating than "normal" fatigue that is typically caused by lack of sleep. There is a validated scale (developed by doctors and submitted to the Journal of Pain and Symptom Management 2000) that assesses CRF on three levels: physical, affective and cognitive subscales. CRF is not relieved by getting more sleep. CRF can last from a few months after chemotherapy or persist for several years after (up to 10 years in some reports). It causes a disruption in every aspect of life: physical, mental, emotional, and psychological.

CRF wreaked havoc on me before I could even define it. I knew I was extremely tired. I was merely calling it 'real tired,' as I had no name for it during my introduction to the problem. I began to call her, *The Beast*! She was a bad-ass, but I was a bigger bad-ass.

My initial encounter with *The Beast* was evident two days after my first round of chemo. My fatigue crept ever so slowly into my life and to date; it seems to have never left; really. I am being honest. As I write this book, I still have moments where I am just drained after moderate exertion. I have to admit that I am not sure if it is CRF or just aging or a combination of the two. Nonetheless, I do not have the stamina I had prior to going through chemotherapy—plain and simple. I believe my body is forever altered due to my breast cancer, chemotherapy and radiation.

On day one post chemo round one, I noticed that I was feeling just a bit tired. I described it in my journal as feeling like I had done a moderately heavy workout and had to push myself to get through the last sets. Little did I know or would eventually come to realize, that I would be feeling like this, times twenty by the end of round four of chemo. I persevered through my 'tiredness' of day one post chemo Round one because I believed that I would be able to get through this with the help of God, My Tribe and my sheer will in honor of all those that had done this (and so many more rounds than my mere four rounds) before me. After all, I had been rehearsing all my life for a time when I had to dig deep, stay focused and persevere. I thought about my parents and their work ethics to stick with things until the end. I thought about Coach Yow and my Mentor Amelia and their perseverance. I was in the battle to win it!

AFTER ROUND ONE OF CHEMO

Days one and two post chemo round one were uneventful, relatively speaking. But soon reality kicked in. *The Beast* was real, as real as the sun sets and the moon rises. The tiredness fully gripped me on day three post chemo round one and it did not relinquish the grip until day nine. I was more than extremely tired. I was asking myself, "Self, I said, how are you going to make it through four rounds of chemo?" At the time, I had no answer, only hope that the chemo would kill the cancer cells that had taken up residence in by right breast and that my life would get back to something that I was familiar with.

When I awoke on day three post chemo of round one, my body felt like it had a large piece of concrete from the highway overpass placed across me. Any movement was deliberate and exhausting. I had to get up to prepare for my workday. *The Beast* was holding me captive on my bed. I just prayed and asked for strength to sit up in the bed. When I sat up, I asked for strength to get out of the bed. Then I got out of bed. I then asked for strength to get to the bathroom. I made it to the bathroom. I just kept asking for strength to move forward. It was more than exhausting. I predicted that I would have some difficulty working if this level of fatigue persisted.

Throughout round one, I persevered each day. Praying and pushing myself to stay in my routine for my semblance of normalcy. I cannot tell you how hard that first bout of tiredness was for me. I knew I had to find a remedy to combat it, as I needed to be functional from day to day.

MIND AND BODY

At the same time the fatigue was weighing on me, it was important to me to maintain some semblance of a schedule that I had prior to the diagnosis. That included a good bed stretch before I got out of bed, a twenty-minute brisk walk, more deliberate stretching and weightlifting daily.

During round one, I was strong enough to do my morning stretches to keep my flexibility—I did not want that to be lost, as I had worked hard to keep my hamstring and quads stretched to reduce any back problems.

Looking back in my journal notes, I wrote that I did a workout or moved (i.e., stretched or lifted weights) every day during all of my chemo rounds; albeit slowly, but I maintained a sense of order for my workout routine to keep me physically fit and moving. I did not want to have a look of sickliness or illness and THEN, have to begin to explain to people why I looked the way I did. If I did not walk each day during this first round, I would bike for ten to fifteen minutes as a substitute. The bike was stationary, and my pace was slow but steady as I watched videos of my YouTube Influencer Friend and Tribe Member Angela.

My physical well-being was essential, and it contributed heavily to my mental well-being. Not being able to ambulate or move around independently meant that I would have to depend on someone else AND I would not be able to do my online work of speech therapy. Staying independent was vital for me and for some reason; it was my raison d'etre (reason for being). I had to survive this journey so that I could share with others and help them too! This determination to thrive and survive the chemo was not new to me; I had seen it done by my parents in their daily lives and in friends and family who had also been on a cancer journey. I needed to make certain that I had enough stamina to do things for myself.

PRAYER THROUGH A PANDEMIC

Remember, a pandemic was happening. In the Middle East, strict rules and regulations were in place to quell the spread. During the early stages of the pandemic due to COVID-19, no one was allowed to mix and mingle in the Middle East. If I had allowed myself to be in need of assistance, I am not sure how that would have played out; a low immune system being subjected to someone else's exposure, could have been detrimental to my well-being. Restrictions in the Middle East prohibited people from mixing and mingling if they were not of the same family. Early on during the pandemic, there were curfews. You were allowed out of your house but only at certain times of the day and you had to stay within your district boundaries, as police cars patrolled the area and checked to be certain you did not stray too far from your district in your quest for food, pharmaceutical needs or anything else. This Middle Eastern country was taking the pandemic very seriously. I was too!

I cannot begin to tell you how many times I asked Mary, Mother of God, for intercession for strength to get through my fatigue hour by hour during round one. My prayers were received, and I was granted mercy by my Lord Jesus Christ, day in and day out throughout my journey. I am so grateful for a merciful God.

My energy levels were low from days three to sixteen post chemo round one. On the sixteenth day post chemo, I wrote in my journal, "Today, a good level of energy—might be steroids (I was taking steroid for my allergic reaction)." I was able to go and do some errands on that day—thank God. After several days of fatigue during round one, all of a sudden, I began to feel as if I had a second wind. Kinda like a runner's kick when you are running a race; you shift into overdrive and bring it home to the finish line. The only problem was the finish line was actually the starting line for round two of chemo and the fatigue would start again and have a different face that would be bigger and badder than the last round.

What I figured out was, by the time I began feeling better and my energy level would allow me to not need as many naps as I had been taking, the next round of chemo would be upcoming. In reading online, some chemo patients reported that the CRF had a cumulative effect; meaning it became more intensified after each round. I had to devise a plan to combat *The Beast* from overtaking my life when she made a return visit for round two.

I was grateful that round one was done, and the fatigue was managed as best I could. On to round two to find what *The Beast* had up her sleeve for me. My second Round was scheduled for four days after my sixteenth day post chemo round one. I prayed that I would be able to handle *The Beast*, who may be bigger and stronger this next round. But first I had to determine whether or not the cooling cap was serving my needs.

Ronnie's Words of Wisdom

There was so much to think about after my first round of chemo. The fatigue was foremost in my mind. I had to learn that when I was tired to nap if time allowed. Naps always refreshed me. Take a nap if you need to, get to know what works best for your body.

NOT SO SURE ABOUT THE COOLING CAP

Fast forward almost three weeks after round one; a few days before my scheduled round two of chemo. My body had been absorbing the chemo drugs and I prayed they were killing the cancer cells in my right breast. I was having some difficulties with allergic reactions, but I was determined and moving forward.

So, picture this: I am in the shower. I pour the shampoo in my hand from the bottle and began to lather my head, as I have always done, rather vigorously. This time, clumps of hair come out! Ohhh...my God...no! I gently washed the soap out and finished bathing. I got out of the shower, dried off and looked in the mirror.

If my Momma were describing what I looked like she would have said I looked "picked headed" meaning I had spots of baldness all over my head. It was a literal mess. I thought to myself: "Self, I said, so much for the cooling cap that was supposed to allow you to keep about 50% of your hair." It had not been a full three weeks and my hair was coming out! Thank God for head scarves being part of the acceptable attire in the Middle East. I was more disappointed than panicked.

With my balding head I tried to comb, ever so gently and style, what little hair I had left. It looked like someone played a board game on my head and shaved all the quasi-squares where they had played. I chuckled to myself! It was a hot mess. But I wrapped it up and no one suspected anything.

In all honesty, I do not believe the cooling cap was functioning properly for me. As I said, my hair did not have icicles in it after the procedure nor did it ever get really cold like I had read and seen on videos. My realization was that my hair was going to fall out and I needed a plan to combat the baldness. But first I would go with it for round two and see what the hair loss was going to be like.

Ronnie's Words of Wisdom

I had no time to think about hair loss. It was somewhat inevitable that I would be losing my hair. That was the least of my worries at this point in the game. I had to gear up for round two and get ready to battle the fatigue.

CHAPTER NINE

Round Two of Chemo

Halfway There!

MY ROUND TWO of chemo was complicated by my various maladies. I developed mucositis, the inflammation of the mucosal (mouth) region, I mentioned previously when discussing oral hygiene. My mouth became really sore. I also had severe itching from one of the cancer drugs. My legs began hurting and feeling heavy with a full feeling that made it seem like they were a chore to lift. I did not have a good gait (walking stride); I often tripped on my marble floors in my flat when nothing was there; it was just me not getting a signal to pick up my feet. This was the beginning of my neuropathy (tingling, pain, decreased sensation in the fingers, feet, and toes). Adding to that in round two, my skin was breaking down. I would later find out that I was allergic to the drug pertusamab, and it would eventually be eliminated from my cocktail. The skin on my neck, chest and back would be on fire with intense itching—cortisone did not help—Zyrtec gave me some relief. I was unable to wear a bra. The areas on my chest and back and under my breasts were so tender and itchy. I was grateful for my Tribe Member, Jen, for sending me some nice camisoles made by Duluth with good strong shelf-bra support that could be worn instead of a bra. My boobs still looked presentable and not just like a pillow across my chest. A definite lifesaving piece of apparel.

On the drive to the hospital for round two, I was feeling tired and prayed that I would get a parking space close to the entrance where I needed to enter the Oncology area. As I rounded the corner near the hospital, I said out loud, "Where is my parking place?" It was an old trick I learned about the power of positive thinking—it worked! A space not far from the entrance was available. I wheeled in and parked. I thanked God for the space and asked for strength to walk to the Center for my treatment. I found myself saying a myriad of little prayers on my walks to my treatments. I just needed that feeling of letting God know I was going in and that he needed to be with me. He never let me down.

I was grappling with an allergic reaction to one of the chemo drugs. Dr. Elyas, my Oncologist was somewhat baffled as to why I had no drug reaction during the administration of round one with any of the drugs, but then later had an itching reaction. It made it difficult for him to discern what drug to eliminate from round two to prevent further allergic reactions. I hoped to find the culprit soon.

Overall, round two was very similar to round one, as I knew what to expect. And I did not do the cooling cap so that made it faster.

For round two, I reported to the Oncology area at 9:00 a.m. for a 9:30 a.m. admission. I got my paperwork, found my room and settled in. Because I knew the routine, I brought some work to do while I had the round of chemo.

For round two, the administration of the chemo drugs went very much like round one; however, the time frame was faster, as they made the drip a bit faster because I was not having an immediate reaction. It still took a while for the drugs to come from pharmacy, but I did not fret about how long it would take. I think I may have even dozed off during the wait.

It was the same routine: get the numbing cream and wait, clean the port area, flush out the port, prep the drugs, and begin the drips. I was still getting both IV drugs, as the Oncologist could not determine which drug was the culprit for the itching. I had no reaction with any of the drips while I was in the Oncology area that day. I got my "hot shot" and waited for any reaction and left about 2:30 p.m. It all took about five hours. I had time to get home, have a nap and see a few clients in the late afternoon then eat something and rest. I was so looking forward to the weekend.

Ronnie's Words of Wisdom

Driving home from round two, I was tired, but I looked forward to falling into bed for a good hour and a half nap before my online sessions. The naps after chemo were always deep and seemed to refresh me. They were just what I needed to present as an upbeat and engaged Speech Therapist to my children online. Some days, the children energized me with their level of enthusiasm and curiosity. I always enjoyed moments when my children had a response that made me laugh. During those times, I was not focused on chemo, but on helping my children have good communication skills. Try to maintain your "typical" schedule if you can; it can allow you some time to NOT focus on your cancer journey; and this can be very healing. It was for me.

AFTER ROUND TWO

Days one through five, post chemo, round two, suckered me and had me thinking "Aw... I got this, *The Beast* ain't got nothin' on me—I got this." I was tired, but not like I was during round one.

Alas, on day six, post chemo, *The Beast* reared her head and tried to bring me down. I persevered. I had read that some vitamin B6 and B12 could help with energy level. That morning, I took about 1000mg of each and hoped for the best. By noon, I was still moving like I was stuck in molasses. I had done additional reading and had found ginseng tablets could be helpful with CRF and I had bought some. I could feel a slight decrease in my level of fatigue. The ginseng did not take away the fatigue, as it lingered and would wash over me intermittently during the day. I felt more tired than any of the other days during round one. Round two, post chemo, was different.

In addition to the fatigue, in round two, I was not sleeping well, and I was getting constipated. So constipated that I had bleeding hemorrhoids. This part may be a bit graphic, but I want you to fully understand the importance of not getting constipated during chemo.

The source of my constipation were the drugs I was taking. My chemo drugs depleted water from my body. This caused my stool (feces) to not be able to move along in my intestine. Moisture (water) is needed for your stool to move along in the digestive tract. The anti-nausea medications that I took had the same effect on my elimination. Even though I drank enormous amounts of water during my chemo and ate a high fiber diet, it was evidently not enough to keep my bowels open and moving. I drank various concoctions that were promoted to help with constipation, but I fell to the culprit of constipation. I was surprised when I first began to have difficulty with my bowels. I did all the things the cancer Counselor had told me to do: drink plenty of water, get exercise, eat leafy greens, and fiber filled vegetables—still constipation started to affect me at the end of round one of my chemo and continued throughout round four until I found a combination that gave me relief. My constipation was so bad, that I had medium sized bleeding hemorrhoids that caused more pain and discomfort than the constipation itself. My diet was high in fiber; I was eating fibrous foods, like Raisin Bran, broccoli, spinach, apples, and raisins; and drinking large amounts of water. Still, I had severe constipation. I was even taking Miralax and having very minimal bowel movements. Constipation made me feel and look bloated and it zapped my energy. I did not need my energy zapped, as I was already running on empty with my CRF. I told my Oncologist about my problem, and he was somewhat baffled and suggested that I try dried figs followed by a glass of water. The figs gave me no relief. The constipation persisted. The Oncologist later recommended a stool softener that had no taste, but the texture and weight of the liquid was like thick mucus. It was rather gross. Thank God it had no taste. I decided that nighttime would be best to try the softener. I mustered enough strength and courage to take two dose caps of the liquid and chased it with water; I went to bed and said a prayer that it would open my bowels. The next morning after my cup of coffee, I got results. I was relieved! I continued with my regime of ample water and leafy greens, fibrous veggies, but nightly I had a double dose of the softener. I finally found the right balance of foods, stool softener, exercise and water that got my bowels back on schedule and managed the constipation.

Ronnie's Words of Wisdom

Ask your doctor for a stool softener. You will have to determine the best dosage for your level of constipation. I needed double doses of stool softener in the beginning, but later I could have good results with a single dose followed by a large glass of warm water. For me, the stool softener worked best if I drank it at night before bed. When I got up the next morning, did my stretches/workout and had my coffee, I was ready to eliminate easily without forcing the process. Having constipation inflicted a glitch in my schedule, as I was accustomed to being on a regular schedule. Once I got the dose of stool softener right for me, I could supplement my diet with healthy fibrous foods that would help with my elimination. Drinking plenty of water was beneficial in combating constipation, not to mention, drinking water is just good for you!

The constipation was the least of my worries. The heavy fatigue in round two went from day six through day nine. The journal entries read that I took naps between my sessions. I look back now and I have to smile that I could awaken from a nap turn on the computer, log into Zoom put on my best animated face and jovial voice for thirty minutes or an hour and do my online session with a little child and then go and collapse into my bed for another thirty or forty-five minute nap, only to get up and do the same thing all over again. How did I do it? Well, my God is an awesome God who willed THAT to happen during this journey—ever soooo grateful for the strength each day, just to get up and move about due to His grace and mercy! Amen!

Post chemo, round two, only prepped me for what was going to happen in round three. Round three was scheduled twenty days after round two.

SHAVING MY HEAD!

My hair loss continued in round two. More and more patches came out each day in the shower and as I combed my hair. It was looking really patchy, but I had a tuft of hair right in the middle of the front part of my head that allowed me to put my scarf just on the hairline so that it appeared like my hair was slicked back under the head wrap. That little tuft of hair would stay with me until the end of round three of chemo. Who was gonna know that I was almost bald?

The weekend pending round three, I went to the hardware store, somewhat similar to Home Depot or Circuit City, here in the Middle East and found beard clippers. I was looking for something to shave my head cleanly so I could wear a skullcap and keep my head wrapped. I found a nice inexpensive set of Baby Bliss clippers with attachments. Once home, I charged them up for a late-night shaving session. I was gonna shave my head! I was desperate to cut off the hair that remained, as it was so patchy and looked hideous.

But first, I needed guidance on how best to shave my head. I had seen my Momma give shape-ups with her manual clippers in her beauty shop years ago, but I was going to shave my entire head. I needed some help.

I video Messengered Pam, my cosmetologist. She was at home in Florida and had gone through her cancer journey years ago. I let her know my plan. I asked her for tips on how to avoid a mess. After a couple of "Gurl, you sure you ready to do it?" questions and some directions I told her I would call her back when I finished. With the clippers charged, and my mirrors ready, the buzzing began.

I had a flashback to when I did this very procedure for my Best Friend, Cynt, years ago. Cynt had been diagnosed with lung cancer that eventually went to her breast and later her brain and she died. I never thought I would be doing it for myself during a pandemic some twenty plus years later in a Middle Eastern country—alone.

It only took a few passes of the shaver to get a bald head as there was not a lot of hair left after two chemo rounds. I had just a bit of stubble that felt funny when I brushed my hand across it. All my hair was gone, and I would now have to wear a skull cap and a head wrap to keep it hidden.

I felt a sense of freedom. I WAS A BALD-HEADED WOMAN and I loved it! I had a heightened sensitivity for air as it swirled around my head when I walked through my flat. I did not really like the feeling of the coolness on my head so I would sleep in the skullcap. My Sister, Edwina. sent me many 'do rags, so I had a nice supply to use for night wear. With the chemo and other drugs, my body became very sensitive to both cold and heat. Since the head keeps in your body heat, I wanted to cover it to help keep warm all the time.

With my new 'do, I video called My Tribe to show off my new look. They were all complimentary and told me that my head shape was a good one for a shaved head. I liked my new look too.

I did not have any feelings of loss for my hair, as I had secretly always wanted short hair all my life. There was no depression or angst about not having hair. I did not want to wear my bald head out, so I wrapped it up as is customary in the Middle East. I embraced my bald head and waited patiently for the day my hair would begin to grow back. I was excited to see what kind of texture and color it would be. My original hair had started to grey, and I had been coloring it to keep the grey at bay. Now, no need for all of that—just a tad bit of shampoo and rinse and some vitamin E oil on my bald dome.

Ronnie's Words of Wisdom

Being bald is fashionable now, but not so much in the Middle East. I am not sure if I would have gone bald had I been in the states. In the Middle East, I covered to avoid questions about my health. You do you—wear your bald head with confidence and flare if that's what you want to do! You are amazing!

CHAPTER TEN

Rounds Three & Four of Chemo

THE CULPRIT FOUND AND FATIGUE ABATED

THIS IS WHEN things started to get really complicated for me. I had to deal with allergic reactions, itching, constipation, mucositis, and the fatigue that had gripped me since round one and was intensifying. Round three of chemo would be a defining moment for me. *The Beast* gained strength during round three. I had battled her pretty well in addition to some other fights along the way, but *The Beast* was uber strong during round three.

The drive to my pre-chemo appointment took a great deal of focus and strength. My fatigue was immense. I parked and as I walked into the hospital my pace was marked by slow and deliberate steps. I had a mantra—"Keep moving forward, you got this, slow and steady," that I repeated until I got to the Oncology department. Then I said a prayer of thanks for making it there; albeit totally wiped out.

I met my Oncologist for pre-chemo round three. I laid out all my ailments and made certain to share about the itching that had persisted even with the help of various anti-itch drugs. They reduced the itching minimally, but it had not subsided. I needed to know what chemo drug was causing the itching. My skin was inflamed, red and bumpy.

When I sat down with Dr. Elyas and he looked at my neck, back and chest and saw my inflamed skin, he was incredulous. He shared that he had grappled with which drug to eliminate. He had decided to forego pertusamab this round as it was the probable culprit for the itching. The elimination of that drug would have the least effect for fighting my cancer. I still had the big guns of docetaxel and the trastuzumab battling it out for me. I was prayerful that during round three my itching would be gone.

During this pre-chemo visit I also shared with Dr. Elyas my concern about the fatigue, as it was getting to be more draining. I told him, that unlike Middle Eastern women who have cancer, they may not be working. I, on the other hand, needed to work for my livelihood, as it was just me.

The day came for round three and it was as expected, sans pertuzumab. My port was cleaned and flushed, and the docetaxel was given via IV. Trastuzumab was given via the controlled injection. No reactions. I was in and out of the Chemo area in about four hours even with the wait for the drugs. I said prayers on the drive home that my itching would stop and that I would be able to combat the fatigue. I was hopeful that the pertusamab was the culprit.

During round three, the fatigue gripped me from day one post chemo until day nineteen. This round, the CRF was not only making me very fatigued, but it was affecting my vision. I had blurred vision and a sty in my eye that was not helping matters. The CRF was making me so tired, that my gait was unsteady. I was not feeling my feet and I would stumble. The chemo-induced neuropathy was setting in.

Ronnie's Words of Wisdom

As I re-read my journal notes during this time, I was still referring to the fatigue as being "tired" or "very tired" or I even called some days "low energy days." It would not be until day nine, post chemo of round three that I found the name of my fatigue— Cancer Related Fatigue (CRF) and gave her the fitting name of *The Beast*. She was relentless and hell-bent on making me feel tired as heck. This round three, *The Beast* would wash over me for several days. It lasted longer than the other two rounds. On day twelve, post chemo round three, my entry reads in all caps: FATIGUE IS LESSENED BUT STILL APPARENT—I AM GRATEFUL.

I had always shared with the medical team my concerns about my fatigue. It was foremost on my agenda, as you know I HAD to work. I was not afforded the luxury of an assistant, maid or anything of that nature to help me with my daily tasks. I had to work for my livelihood. The idea of having to deal with a double dose of fatigue had me thinking that I would have to cancel my therapy sessions with my clients. My client's parents would begin to wonder what was happening with their level of service. I needed a remedy for *The Beast* if she was gonna double team me with round four coming in a few days.

When I met with Dr. Elyas for my pre-chemo round four, I told him that the fatigue seemed to go longer in round three than in round two, and if round four was in a few days, that I would not be certain that I could still work. During days fifteen through seventeen of round three, I was Googling "remedies for CRF." I told him about the research I found by the National Institutes of Health (NIH). The study used the drug methylphenidate, the active ingredient in an attention deficit hyperactivity disorder (ADHD) to help with fatigue in cancer patients. Methylphenidate acts to increase the level of dopamine in the central nervous system. Dopamine makes you feel good. In the study, the evidence for the efficacy of its use was weak. However, the patients reported that they felt better when they took the drug. Eureka! That is all the evidence I needed. I pleaded my case on top of looking totally washed out and just plain whooped. Even the Oncologist could see how fatigued and slow moving I was. Dr. Elyas was amenable to trying the drug after his intern checked for any medical contraindications with my current drug regime.

They wrote a prescription for Concerta for me to get it at the pharmacy. I would have the drug before my next round of chemo and prayerfully feel better.

When I got to the pharmacy, there was a problem with the paperwork. The drug was considered a controlled substance in the Middle East and had to have additional paperwork in order for me to get it. I was exhausted from my appointment, and I chose to return the next day when the paperwork had been completed. I had to go home and rest and prep for an online session. I was praying that Concerta would be my holy grail.

The next day I returned to the pharmacy. I presented my information for the release of the drug and was able to get the Concerta, as it was approved and paid for by my insurance.

I drove back home, read the instructions, which included a statement that the drug was highly addictive. I knew that I did not need an addiction problem on top of the cancer, and I told myself that I would only use the Concerta on the days when my energy level was so low that I could not muster up energy to get through the day.

I was still reeling from *The Beast* on day 20 post chemo round three. I wanted to see what the effects of Concerta were so, I took the Concerta on a Friday morning (as a trial) with a small finger sandwich. You had to take it with food. I wanted to see the effects of it so that I would know if it was effective for me to get through my days.

When I tell you Concerta, for me, was a game changer, I am not doing the drug justice. I was able to push through my day with one nap and not feel like I was devastated. I had evenness with my energy level. I likened it to a fine-tuned car, just running smoothly and pushing forward with no added extra effort. I was just humming along during my day. That is what Concerta did for me. I felt like I could overtake *The Beast*. But at 6:00 p.m., I was wiped out. Concerta is time released and it only stays in your system a certain amount of time and then it is out. I was very pleased with the level of energy I had with the Concerta in my trial. I was armed and ready for *The Beast* in round four. Round four of chemo came twenty-one days after round three.

ROUND FOUR OF CHEMOTHERAPY: BEATING *THE BEAST*

I was so tired from round three. *The Beast* along with the constipation had zapped all my energy. It was comforting to know that I had the Concerta just waiting for the moment when *The Beast* reared her head. What was even more satisfying was knowing I was at the end of my mandatory four rounds of chemo for the neoadjuvant protocol (chemo first, with hopes the tumor shrinks, then surgery, then radiation). I achieved my milestone! Now, I could prepare to move to the next step of the process: repeated ultrasound, MRI, and CT scans to determine if the tumor had shrunk or had been eliminated.

Ronnie's Words of Wisdom

It is imperative to keep moving forward in your journey. As always, at the start, I did not know what my finish line looked like, but I did know that day by day I would make forward progress so that I positioned myself to see the end on the horizon. Push forward, you know the end is out there—this is your epitome of the definition of faith—"the realization of what is hoped for; the evidence of things unseen" (Hebrews 11:1)—Be faithful and believe.

On my final drive to my last round of chemo I not only thought about how drained I was but how I would be free from the fatigue at some point soon. Without the drugs causing the fatigue surely, I would be on the road to having my energy level return. I ran a quick little vignette of a vibrant, happy, energetic Ronnie in my head and smiled. I turned to my prayers of gratitude for getting through all the rounds, for being able to drive myself to my appointments, and for continuing to work each day. I was grateful for God's mercy. Just writing this down makes it seem like it is something out of storybook, but it is what I overcame in my cancer journey. I learned to embrace this, my victory. Finishing the four rounds of chemo meant that I was winning, and I was going to beat whatever challenge(s) came next. That was my motivation to keep on keeping on.

Round four went very much like round three, and once again I was in and out of the Oncology area in about four hours total. I was so grateful for getting through my four rounds of chemo. Though I did not look forward to the cumulative effects of what round four would bring.

Days one and two and post chemo, round four were ok. Not very tiring. I had other battles with constipation and eyesight, but I was not overly tired like after my other rounds. I was able to keep moving forward.

Day three, post chemo, round four—the fatigue was beginning to wash over me. I would start to do something in the flat like wash clothes and just become exhausted from gathering the clothes to put them in the washer. I knew *The Beast* was lurking. Late in the evening that day, I got really tired—that was weird, as I had not previously had any fatigue at night. My fatigue typically was during the day. I thought to myself: "Self, I said, *The Beast* is going to show up tomorrow." I was grateful that I had something for the counterattack—Concerta. I would assess my fatigue the next morning and decide if I needed to have a tablet to get through my day. I told myself—"if needed, tomorrow you will bring out the Concerta and fight *The Beast*."

Day four, post chemo, round four was after a restless night of sleeping (this was another strange phenomenon that happened; I typically slept through the night—*The Beast* was lying in wait). I woke up to the feeling of that concrete slab lying on me and I felt incapacitated. I had body pain and I felt like someone had been punching me. Without hesitation, I took the Concerta. I had a small sandwich with it and chugged a glass of water. I went about my morning routine of stretching and exercising and getting ready for the day. I was moving through my day! The Concerta gave me control over *The Beast*. I was functional. I went through my day with a nap, not several. I managed to see all of my clients. I was able to overtake *The Beast* on this day four, post chemo of round four. I did not want to celebrate too long, as the next day was coming, and I did not know what lay in store for me.

I took Concerta on days four through seven, and later on days ten and eleven of round four chemo. I did not need the Concerta on the other days; my CRF was manageable with my sheer will to persevere. I had made a pact with myself that I would only use the Concerta on the days when my CRF was so bad in relation to the level of my functionality. I stuck with it. I was prescribed twenty-eight tablets, and I took only seven.

I am so thankful I did my research to find this drug to help with my CRF. It was a lifesaver for me. It is hard to describe how the Concerta pushed me through my day. I remember thinking I am like the *Little Train That Could*. I would do one thing and not feel exhausted and another with the same feeling. Before I knew it, I had done a whole lot of things without a flicker of a feeling of exhaustion. Most importantly, I had energy to do my online sessions in an upbeat spirit and not feel totally drained after thirty minutes. That was pleasant and welcomed after round four. I was grateful for finding out about the effects of the Concerta. I was blessed that I persevered and that my Oncologist was open to an alternative to combat the CRF.

Ronnie's Words of Wisdom

I thought about my Momma who problem solved—I channeled her in finding a remedy for my fatigue.

Did I mention the itching stopped too? Eliminating the pertuzumab was the right decision for me. It took my skin awhile to clear up, but OMG, was I glad that I was not itching. I was a very pleased patient, itch-free and had energy.

The overall chemo journey was nothing short of a good detective story like a "Who Dunnit?" I am grateful I had a Doctor who was willing to listen to my concerns and would try something that was outside the protocol to help with the fatigue. I would tell him later that he should be prescribing Concerta for all his patients who suffer from CRF and he was in agreement.

Now, chemo was done. I had to wait about four weeks until I could have the ultrasound, mammogram, MRI and CT tests repeated. All my doctors were hoping for a positive/complete clinical response (P/CCR), meaning that the tumor would shrink or be resolved (disappear) as a result of the chemo. I prayed I would be healed, if it were God's will and was hopeful the drugs had done what they were supposed to do. The rest was in God's hands.

Next steps, I made my appointments for a repeat ultrasound, mammogram, MRI and CT scan so that those images could be compared to the initial ones taken at the beginning of the journey. Then I had an Oncology appointment scheduled, to get my Herceptin subcutaneous injection to fight the receptors in my body and stop them from making the protein that the cancer found nourishing. I would have seventeen total injections of Herceptin per protocol to keep my cancer at bay. Now back to the waiting game.

Ronnie's Words of Wisdom

My rounds of chemo were the biggest challenge in my journey, heck, my life. While daunting, chemo is not impossible to get through. I kept myself motivated by prayer, with My Tribe and thinking of my friends, family and Mentors who had done far more rounds of chemo than my mere four. They had demonstrated strength and perseverance in their fight. I wanted to have the same grit. I stayed in the moment and celebrated my victories, driving myself to and from each of my chemo appointments, eating right, getting naps. Keep moving forward in your journey. Every step forward is getting you closer to beating your challenge. You will find, as I did, that you have a deep level of fight in your very being that will rise to the occasion. You got this!

CHAPTER ELEVEN

A Different Kind of Round

Trastuzumab Meet Denosumab

HAVING COMPLETED FOUR rounds of chemotherapy was a reason to celebrate; but my jubilance was always short-lived, for I knew there were more procedures, medications, and appointments to come. Chemotherapy was tremendously hard, not because I had to drive myself to my sessions, but because of the physical, mental, emotional and spiritual strain it caused. My body was battered, but I knew I needed to garner strength to keep up the fight. My thoughts shifted to all the people I had known who had fought their own battles. People like my Mentor—Amelia, my Momma, and my Aunt Elsie, and my former Coach Kay Yow all who did far more rounds of chemo than my measly four. My rounds were hard, but what they went through was far more difficult and they each fought hard to the very end. I channeled their courage daily.

With chemo in my rear-view mirror, I still had a long road ahead of me with my trastuzumab injections. I had to get seventeen rounds. This drug would continue to fight against those proteins that my body made that the cancer fed on. I had completed four trastuzumab injections along with my chemo rounds.

Ronnie's Words of Wisdom

The cancer journey is just that, a journey. Many twists and turns along a very long road. You catch glimpses of the destination but there is always a road sign that pops up and has you make a detour, prolonging your trip. I ended up gaining my patience and perseverance wings. I learned about the present and being in it in the moment and got comfortable with just waiting. Deep breaths- you got this!

To get my remaining rounds of trastuzumab, I would set up an appointment with my Oncologist on the fifteenth day after the last injection. The injections needed to be every twenty-one days. I still had a way to go. I continued my schedule on Thursdays, as that day would give me the weekend to recuperate. There were really no side effects of the trastuzumab. My CRF continued to linger and dominate my life, long after my four rounds of chemo were done and even after my seventeenth round of trastuzumab.

Ronnie's Words of Wisdom

To continue to take the Concerta to combat the CRF was not an option for me. Concerta is a highly addictive drug, and I didn't want an addiction added to my life. I exercised discipline and did not use the remaining Concerta tablets. What I did was keep a solid schedule, take naps when I got fatigued, eat healthy foods with lots of protein, limit my carbs, and continue to work out daily to keep up my strength. Even as I write this book, I have continued to manage my CRF. Sometimes, I wonder if it is CRF or merely the aging process taking over. Nonetheless, I will keep moving forward and be grateful for each day, as you will too in your cancer journey.

A NEW DRUG

The schedule of Oncology appointments and injections continued for thirteen sessions after my last chemo. During round eight of trastuzumab, a new drug was introduced into the mix.

As I mentioned before, there are a plethora of tests that are done before each round of chemo and prior to the trastuzumab injections. It is important for the Oncologist to know my liver function levels, CBC (complete blood count) levels, vitamin D levels, and bone profile measures prior to administering doses of drugs. Every twenty-one days these levels were taken via blood samples. It was determined that my calcium levels were low, and I needed a drug to boost those levels. Denosumab was added in round eight along with the trastuzumab injections. The good thing about Denosumab was that I only had to have that injection every six months. I would add that drug to my list in *My Appointment Notebook* and track the progress. I was later told that even after I am finished with everything, I would still have the Denosumab injections to combat any osteopenia (brittle bones) that may develop from aging and from the long-term effects of the chemo drugs.

In general, the trastuzumab and Denosumab injections were a breeze. I began to view anything that was not chemotherapy as easy. To this day, chemotherapy remains THE hardest thing that tested my fortitude.

On 21 October 2021, one year and thirteen days after my first round of chemo, I did my last trastuzumab injection. It is customary to bring a gift of some kind to the staff in appreciation for the level of care received. I brought the Medical Staff in the Oncology area some ma'amoul (a delicious date cookie) from my friend Tina. Her shop is a French Patisserie Shoppe, *Sucré Salé*. I purchased some glass containers with lids and placed some ma'amoul in each container and labeled it with their name and a note of thanks. I was truly grateful for the level of care that the staff had provided for me during my rounds of chemo and trastuzumab. Though we were celebrating the end of the fourteen sessions, I would still see them every six months for the Denosumab injection for the next five years. I was in for the duration of this process.

Ronnie's Words of Wisdom

The typical protocol for post chemo treatment is five years from the date you are diagnosed. Right after completing the rounds of chemo there are tests to determine the status of the cancer. If those tests are clear, they are repeated in six months. Then if those follow up test results are clear and cancer free, the protocol calls for annual checkups for the next five years. If after five years there are no signs of cancer (complete remission), then you are deemed cancer-free. This became my new goal.

After blessing the Oncology area staff with their gifts, I made my way to the Oncology department to give the staff there my tokens of appreciation. I had gotten date loaves from *Sucré Salé* to share with the medical team. I chatted with my Oncologist and the staff and thanked them all for the excellent level of care I had received.

Now it was time to shift back to the next steps in the sequence— repetition of the ultrasound, mammogram, MRI, and CT scan. With God, and My Tribe I forged on.

ALL CLEAR AFTER CHEMO

Fast forward four weeks after my chemo was completed. I had my ultrasound, mammogram, MRI and CT repeated and was anxiously awaiting news of the condition of the tumor—was it gone? smaller? Along with My Tribe, I had prayed for healing, but we always added, "May God's will be done." I now know that secretly they were praying that the cancer would be eliminated and that I would have more time here with them. I was praying for the same thing; it was my human response. This experience confirmed for me that when I got through this ordeal, I would share all that I learned and the various tricks to navigate a cancer diagnosis. I knew I was going to share my experience with others no matter the outcome. Ideally, I wanted more time to get my story told, so I could help others like me and help their Tribes.

I received a call from my Breast Surgeon, Dr. Rena. She was usually so cheerful, but this time her voice had a lilt that sounded happy and joyous. She said, "Veronica, My Dear, you had what we call a positive clinical response to chemo—the tumor was eliminated." I contained my excitement and shifted into my intellectual response mode. I would have lost it at this point if I allowed myself to get emotional. I needed to get information and I needed to stay attentive to the matter at hand.

Ronnie's Words of Wisdom

As I type this, I am crying and feeling very blessed about the outcome of my chemo. Putting it on paper has me reliving the call and shifting completely to my emotional response. I still remember the feeling of gratefulness that I had at that moment. I am and will always be truly blessed.

In my intellectual response mode, I said: "Alhumdulilallah" Arabic translated is (God's blessing be upon it). Dr. Rena agreed, "Yes, Alhumdulilallah." The next words out of my mouth were: "What's the next step? Can we schedule the surgery?" Dr. Rena knew me at this point and was not surprised that I did not want to dwell on the moment. Instead, I was ready to prepare for the next step in the process. Dr. Rena replied, "Come for a follow-up appointment and we can discuss the surgical plan." After the call ended, I scheduled the next available date, which was just a few days away.

The follow-up meeting with Dr. Rena was long, about forty minutes. I really wanted to understand what she was sharing with me about my complete clinical response to chemotherapy. It was a "hats off" moment for the Tumor Board in their recommendation to do the neoadjuvant approach rather the adjuvant approach with the surgery first. They had achieved the goal of destroying the tumor, making it less likely to have cancer cells remaining near it, if it had merely been shrunk.

When Dr. Rena brought up my new MRI, CT, mammogram, and ultrasound images in a side-by-side panel on her computer, it was amazing to see the difference in the lesion (tumor) from the before images, versus the after images. The tumor had vanished. All that remained was the marker. What was even more amazing was when the contrast was done in the image after the chemo, there was not that direct line from my vein to the lesion that was so clear-cut on the previous one. I was silently saying, "My God is an Awesome God."

Then Dr. Rena mentioned the concern the Radiologist had with my left breast, and my heart sank. I thought to myself, "I do have lumpy breasts"—so.... go figure? During the second ultrasound, a mass had been found in my left breast—my thought was "not sure I wanna do a sequel to this show." However, she reassured me by giving me visuals she knew I would comprehend. Dr. Rena went on to explain that the mass had been seen in the first images and there was not a concern, as it did not take up the contrast as the right breast tumor had. I am thinking... yes... that makes sense... but I want to hear more. She went on to say that even if there was a small chance that the mass in my left breast was cancerous, it was not showing signs of being malignant. She then paused and made a very good clarification. Because of my history of breast cancer and familial link (Mother and Aunt), the Radiologist would tend to err on the side of caution and give the breast a BIRADS rating of three and watch it for six months, then repeat the imaging. BIRADS stands for Breast Imaging Reporting Data System. It is a system that categorizes breast images. The categories range from 0 (findings are unclear; more images are needed) to six (cancer was diagnosed using a biopsy). My category of three meant that the findings were probably benign (noncancerous) but needed follow-up in six months. I was ok with this status.

The information Dr. Rena shared was understandable; however, I did not want to take the focus away from my upcoming surgery. I had to stay in the present and get the surgery done to keep moving through the process to get back to a good, healed and healthy body. Dr. Rena all but reassured me that the mass in my left breast was a Fibroadenoma or a benign, solid, not fluid filled lump. I had to ask Dr. Rena a logical question—"Can a Fibroadenoma turn into a cancerous tumor." She repeated it back as if she had it memorized like a school mnemonic device. Then, she responded, "no, it cannot." A wave of relief poured over me as she spoke those words.

I waited for Dr. Rena to call to arrange the day and time for the surgery. At this point in the process, I did not need prior approval. Dr. Rena was able to book my surgery for 17 January 2021. I would have to report to the anesthesia area at 7:30 a.m. I would be one step closer in completing the protocol for the removal of the cancer. It was going to be a big day.

Now my timelines seemed to be moving at a steady pace. It was on December 10, 2020, that I had my last chemo round. Five weeks later, I was preparing for surgical removal of the area where I had a cancerous lump residing in my right breast.

Some of you may ask why have surgery if the lump was resolved? The protocol for breast cancer calls for removal of the area where the lump was called the margins. These margins are typically a rim of tissue around the site anywhere from one to two millimeters in circumference. During my lumpectomy, the tissue taken in the margins at the site will be sent out for testing to ensure that no undetected cancer cells are present. This ensures that all cancer is removed and decreases the chances of reoccurrence. Keep in mind the sentinel node (in my right arm pit) will also be tested during surgery for cancerous cells. This is an excellent surgical method to ensure that cancer does not recur. As another line of defense, after the surgery, I will do some rounds of radiation to ensure no cancer remains at the site. I wanted a healed healthy body. This methodology assured me that all bases were covered. I was blessed.

Ronnie's Words of Wisdom

I was so happy to get this point in my journey. Having the surgery scheduled meant I was closer to beating my cancer. While the journey seemed long, I knew my level of care had been exceptional and for that I was grateful.

CHAPTER TWELVE

The Surgery

My Lumpectomy

AFTER MY VERY thorough meeting with Dr. Rena, I had to think about my surgery. It would be an early morning procedure that would require me to stay overnight in the hospital.

Ronnie's Words of Wisdom

I was feeling optimistic about my pending surgery. I had a level of confidence and rapport with my medical team that was mentally soothing. I was not worried about the surgery, as it had been spelled out to me and I could understand the procedures. I felt my optimism was a sure sign that

> I had come to a reckoning with the fact I would
> undergo surgery to remove whatever remained of
> the tissue from the cancerous site. I was certain I
> had rounded the corner on this cancer journey and
> was preparing to head into the home stretch.

When I told my Tribe, Angela, my friend and also a Registered Nurse working at a hospital in the Eastern region of the Middle East about nine hours from me, volunteered to come and be with me a few days before and after the surgery. It was comforting knowing that she would be with me. I knew she would make sure I would get the level of care that was needed; she would be my Guardian Angel watching over me. It would be a mere plane ride for the visit, and I would be there to pick her up from the airport. The plan was she would arrive a few days before my surgery. She knew the protocol with COVID-19, and I was comforted in her knowledge and the precautions she took on my behalf to care for me.

Ronnie's Words of Wisdom

Let me tell you about friends who will be there for
you no matter what. My Tribe was my "Ride or
Die;" that is, they had my back through this ordeal.
I took solace in knowing that if I called and asked
for anything during this journey they would be
there; plain and simple. You may have friends or a
significant other like this already. If you do not, it
is my prayer that you find a few people who will be
there for you; no questions asked. Find your Tribe.

THE BIG DAY

Finally, the day of the surgery arrived. Bear in mind, my fourth round of chemo had been on December 10, 2020. My post-surgery appointment with Dr. Rena was on December 27th. It was two weeks later, and I was going to have surgery for the removal of the area where the tumor had been in my right breast. I was ready. My fatigue level was ok. I think the excitement of surgery kicked in and my adrenalin was keeping me going.

Angela and I got up early. I had my coffee and did my morning stretches, meditation and prayers. We headed to the hospital, parked and did a short walk to the main building. I had to go to a different area for check in for surgery. Once checked in, Angela was not allowed to be with me. I had my phone and stayed in touch. My other Tribe member Angie would plan to come later in the day. She worked at a nearby hospital. She and Angela would wait for me in recovery and then go with me to my room.

After checking in, I was taken back and given a gown along with those webby panties to change into. I left my clothes and a few personal belongings in the locker provided. I could not take my phone on the gurney, so I sent my last message to My Tribe asking for their continued prayers. My memory is fuzzy on this, but I do recall meeting Dr. Rena, my surgeon and her telling me all was going to be well. I also met several other doctors who would be assisting or observing. I was wheeled to the ultrasound area. They needed to insert a thin wire localization needle for marking the site and guiding the surgeon to ensure that they have the correct spot to remove the tissue. Dr. Rena told me about this procedure. Anesthesia was used to numb my breast and the wire was inserted— it was basically pain free and a low level of discomfort overall. Once that was done, I was headed to the OR (operating room) where I got my real anesthesia (propofol) and off to la-la-land I went.

Ronnie's Words of Wisdom

As I was wheeled off to the surgical area, I prayed Dr. Rena would have a steady hand and perform well. I prayed for the other medical team members that they would perform their jobs well. I had words of gratitude that the tumor disappeared with the chemo, for getting through the chemo, and for my Tribe. I wanted to cry because I was so happy this moment had finally come, but I did not for fear the medical team would interpret the tears as fear—I was overjoyed, and my heart was full of gratitude and love of life. Practice gratitude as much as you can. It will uplift you in your journey.

During the lumpectomy, Dr. Rena would remove the area where the tumor was and remove tissue in a margin around that area to ensure that any remaining and undetected cancer cells were removed. The sample would be sent out during the surgery for testing. I heard of people having clear margins after surgery and now it made perfect sense.

Also, during the lumpectomy, Dr. Rena would be taking a look at my sentinel (first) node under my right arm. This group of the lymph nodes is the first to receive drainage from a tumor. They are removed and tested during the lumpectomy and information is conveyed back if they are positive or negative for cancer. The area of my breast was injected with a methylene blue dye, which had radioactive properties in it. A probe was then used to track the dye to the sentinel node and then Dr. Rena could remove it for testing. After the sample was taken to the lab, we expected results to be back quickly. This information was vital. If the sample was positive, more nodes would have to be removed and tested. The removal of the lymph nodes can mean a life of dealing with lymphedema (swelling in the arm on the side of the site) that can be bothersome and painful. If the sample is negative the area is sutured, and the lumpectomy would continue. My lymph nodes were clear in compliance with the results of the MRI and CT scans from weeks ago. My surgery was about three hours total. I was in recovery before the afternoon. I woke up in my large private room with Angela sitting in the comfy chair nearby and Angie would come later. Then we could Girlfriend!

My hospital room was a traditional private room as was custom in the Middle East. It was divided into an outer area with several sofas along the wall and a coffee table. The sofas converted into beds so family members can stay over and be close to their loved ones. In the next room was my room with the hospital bed and all the monitors necessary. There was a refrigerator, and another area to make coffee or tea. The room came stocked with water, coffee, and tea. It had a very homey vibe. Getting back to my room after recovery, it was nice to see Angela waiting for me. She immediately put on her Nurse's hat and asked about my pain level, whether or not I needed anything, and was I comfortable, etc. It was so nice to have this level of love and care after my surgery.

AFTER THE SURGERY

I had minimal pain after the surgery because the anesthesia was still in my body. I felt ok and a little tired. My lips were dry, and Angela got my lip balm so I could apply a coat on my lips and then drink some water. I drank A LOT of water after surgery. I had fasted since the night before, so I was more than parched.

After all the water, I had to urinate. I was able to get up out of bed with minimal assistance from Angela. She took my IV pole with my antibiotic and pain drip hanging on it alongside me to the bathroom. It felt good to pee. When I finished, I turned to flush and I noticed the water was greenish/bluish and I thought to myself: "Self, I said, they must use a Ty-D-Bol cleaner." I did not think of the color of the water until later when I got home. After about an hour or so of being in my room I was visited by a Dr. Tarek, who had assisted in the surgery. He came to check on me and to look at the site. He was surprised to see me so alert. I was already on my phone searching for stuff. He asked about my pain level, I said about a three out of ten—it was minimal, thank God. When he looked at the site, there was no redness or swelling and just a bit of leakage. He changed the dressing, which allowed Angela to get a picture of the site for me. It was not bad looking. There was just a line at about 9:00 on my right breast. The incision was about one inch and three quarters long. Just a few sutures held it together. The area under my arm had two sutures and Dr. Tarek said they looked fine.

After changing the dressing, Dr. Tarek gave me instructions for bathing. The site had a waterproof bandage on it, so I could get it wet. He told me after three days, to remove the bandage and I could still get it wet, and the steri-strips would eventually fall off when the site was healed. It took about ten days for the last piece of steri-strip to fall off and for the sutures to resolve. It was a nice-looking incision. I kept Bio-Oil and NewGel +E on it nightly and during the day to prevent scarring. To date, it looks like a minimal scar or blemish.

Ronnie's Words of Wisdom

I used Bio-Oil and a silicone gel, NewGel +E, on all my incisions, even on my port incision after it healed. Today it is barely visible with no keloid (thick raised scar). On my breast scar, I had the same results and under my arm at the node site –minimal scarring. All my scars look good and smooth with no edges or ridges or keloids. Get Bio-Oil and silicone gel after your scars heal. Even if you have old scars, Bio-Oil is helpful.

FINALLY, AN OVERNIGHT GUEST

Now, I had to mentally prep for a night in the hospital. It had been a while since I was in a hospital overnight. The last time was when I blew out my Achilles tendon many years prior. It was comforting to have Angela with me. Angie was able to stay a while and we laughed and talked about all kinds of stuff! We even took funny pictures!

Ronnie's Words of Wisdom

Angela and Angie made being in the hospital feel like a staycation. We just vibed together, as we always did with our crazy discussions about various topics and what was happening in our lives. Having my two Tribe members with me gave me such consolation and peace. I did not think about my surgery, they kept me occupied and engaged. I knew that I was in good hands and that I was going

> to have many moments of laughter with lots of
> love. On this journey, it will be your friends who will
> keep you lifted up and help you to keep on keeping
> on. Friends make the journey easier.

They served us lentil soup, rice, chicken, mixed veggies, Arabic bread, cheese, olives and a small salad for dinner. It was pretty good even though I did not eat a lot. One thing is for sure, in the Middle East, you will eat well and healthily.

I was getting tired and prepared for bed. Angela converted her chair into the sleeper lounger and put on her PJs. We both read some and went to bed. I could not sleep because the beeps, bells, alarms went off ALL night long. In addition, the Nurses were coming every few hours for a vital signs check. By morning, I was exhausted and ready to go home and get in my bed. We had to wait for my discharge papers. I had seen Dr. Tarek earlier in the morning and he said all looked well and I could go home "Inshallah" (God willing) before noon. Angela and I were ready to leave. She had rested well and comfy on the lounger, but we were ready to be at my flat and get home comfy.

I got discharged a bit after 1:00 in the afternoon. We packed up and headed home. On the way, I suggested we get seafood bags for our meal. We made a quick detour and went to Shrimp Zone for a couple of bags of shrimp with potatoes and corn and lemon pepper seasonings. We were going to have a feast.

When we arrived at the flat, and made our way over to my door, right away, I knew something was amiss. My door to the outside area was slightly cracked—I did not leave it like that. Someone had been to my flat! As I unlocked the door and entered, I saw the most beautiful purple (my favorite color) orchid on my kitchen counter. My other Tribe member, Sage, had let herself in and left me a lovely plant with a note to get well soon. My Tribe—I love them! Angela and I got settled and began to have our feast. It was delicious. Angela kept asking how I felt, I would respond I was ok. She asked what my pain level was at. I would say about a three. My pain was not bad at any point after the surgery. What was uncomfortable for me was the limited range of motion (ROM) I had in my right arm/ shoulder and chest area. I knew that I would have to alter my stretches and workouts, to avoid separating the sutures or causing pain. I was making my plan in my head on how to adjust my workout the next day.

We washed up what few dishes there were and headed to bed. We did not make plans for the next day, as everything depended on how I would be feeling. I had to sleep on my back, but I rested well. I had practiced this the weeks before, as I anticipated not having use of my right side. I was grateful for a good night's rest. Before retiring for the night, I had to go to the bathroom. After I urinated, the water was green, and I was like, WHOA! I yelled to Angela to come and see. With her Nursing hat on and unfazed, she said they must have given you some dye. I had forgotten about the sentinel node procedure and the use of dye. I was relieved. I thought I had become an alien!

The next day, I got up to do my morning stretches and that's when I realized my ROM was limited. When I did my morning salutation, I could not extend my arms straight up over my head. My right arm had a bend. With my forward fold, I could not fully extend down. I quickly surmised that any of my stretches that required arm extension would be limited, but only for the time being. I made a mental note and stretched as best I could and got through my entire routine.

For me, there was not a great deal of pain after my lumpectomy. What bothered me most was my limited ROM for extending my arms straight up over my head like for a tree pose or doing jumping jacks for my workouts. The first few days after the surgery when I tried to extend my arms up over my head, I felt some tingling sensations in my arms. Each day, I made note of the range I achieved and tried to go a little bit further every day.

I was able to keep my morning routine. Angela had some coffee and we chatted. Like clockwork she asked how I felt, and I told her I felt fine. I suggested we go to the luxury shopping mall so that she could shoot video for @angelamashelle, her YouTube channel. Angela created her channel for women over forty. She provides beauty, fashion and lifestyle content. Without hesitation she was in agreement. We got showered and off we went. I drove, as I was feeling fine.

We went to Jimmy Cho and Angela fell in love with three pairs of shoes. Two were on sale, and one not so much. We went to the Gucci store. Then we went to another luxury mall, but not after making a stop at McDonalds where Angela showed me how she eats French fries and a vanilla ice cream cone—I tasted it, not bad—but weird. On for more shopping. A stop at the Valentino store had Angela buying some cute sandals that she had been looking for. Then we headed home. I was thinking about dinner. I was craving some fish, so we ordered fish and rice for dinner and called it day.

Overall, I felt ok. I was tired but not too tired to shop. My logic was to keep moving and stay in a routine. I did not want my arm to get stiff and lose more of my ROM. My surgery went well. No complications and I healed like a champ. I was happy with my scars;

they were not big, and they healed nicely. Regarding my limited ROM, I ever so slowly would try to extend my arm to get straighter and straighter each day. As a former Division I athlete I knew how to modify my movements to accommodate my ROM. It took about two weeks, and I was fully extending and folding like I had been before. No ROM had been lost in the interim of the surgery!

Ronnie's Words of Wisdom

Sometimes, you just have to keep pushing forward. Your first thought may be to rest, because you have been through this procedure or that procedure but keep moving and stay agile. Ten days later, I was doing my full extensions without any sensations. It was imperative that I stay active and move and stretch daily. I know this heavily contributed to my solid rehabilitation and my ability to overcome cancer in my journey. Move, even if it is just a few steps each day. Day by day, add to those steps and keep yourself moving and mobile—you will be glad you did. Remember: Move it or lose it.

Angela stayed on one more day and we just chilled. I thanked her profusely as we drove back to the airport. It was good to have someone with me during the surgery and after. Even though I had no complications, just the company was good; and company with a Nursing perspective made it even better. I already missed her as I dropped her at the airport. I changed my thought pattern from sadness to gratitude for her, Angie and Sage, and for friends who cared so much.

That afternoon, I was back to my routine. I had my sessions online as scheduled. Still, I did not have pain, nor did I feel sick. I greeted my clients online with a big smile and my head wrapped. I was ready to help them communicate more effectively in their therapy session.

THE FOLLOW-UP

All that was left to do was to have a follow-up appointment with Dr. Rena, my breast surgeon. This happened about ten days after the surgery. I was doing well. The steri-strips were almost off and the incision to me looked well—no swelling, redness or infection. Dr. Rena agreed when she saw the site and thought it was going to be a good scar that would fade eventually. She said it was all good. Next steps would be radiation to irradiate any cancer cells that may have been missed with the chemo. This is called prophylactic (just in case/preventative) treatment. Later, the MRI and CT scans would be repeated in six months to ensure that all the cancer was eliminated. Next up Radiation—a new journey!

CHAPTER THIRTEEN

The Easy Part of Cancer Treatment for Me

Radiation

I COMPLETED MY FOUR rounds of chemotherapy back in early December of 2020 and my lumpectomy on 17 January 2021. I would continue with trastuzumab for thirteen injections as part of the chemo protocol. Time seemed to really be moving along quickly.

Now, I also needed to begin my radiation therapy even though the tumor was reabsorbed (dissolved) during the chemo. God is good AND won't He do it? It is customary protocol to do several rounds of radiation to ensure all the cancer cells are demolished.

Ronnie's Words of Wisdom

Before my radiation I had to call my Oncologist and Breast Surgeon when the COVID vaccine became available in the Middle East. They both agreed it would be safe for me, and also that I should get it to try to keep COVID at bay with my compromised immune system. I got the vaccine and luckily had no side effects from it. When you are immune compromised you need to be extra careful.

My Oncologist and Radio-Oncologist scheduled me for fifteen consecutive daily rounds of radiation (weekends not included). I found out In order to provide radiation for cancer patients there needs to be many standards in place with the facility/room that the radiation machine will be placed. Actually, after a deep dive into radiation machines I found that all types of radiation or X-rays required various guidelines for safety. Specially designed doors, walls, ceilings, glass, were required to have a certain thickness, size, material and space for obvious safety and health concerns. The hospital where I received my chemo was unable to provide the radiation as they did not have a room that met the guidelines mentioned above for the type of radiation I needed for the breast cancer.

I had to drive across town to a university teaching hospital to get measured for my radiation treatments. The drive to the hospital was a bear. Parking was a problem and a nightmare, as people parked anywhere and everywhere, often blocking others in. I often thought how many people were there on any given day that required far more treatment than radiation. I counted myself blessed and did not complain. I opted to park in a rather distant "lot" and walk to the hospital. I had to walk very slowly. The hospital sat on a slight uphill grade and the temp was about eighty-two degrees, and the sun was very hot and bright. As I walked uphill to the hospital, I just measured my steps. I used my slow, rhythmic breathing and paced myself. I was exhausted once I arrived at the front desk to check in. My CRF (cancer related fatigue) was still reeling in my body after the chemo. The walk had taken all my energy.

The Radiation department was tucked neatly in a corner that required several twists and turns and attentive reading of signage for directions. Finally, I arrived at the check in desk. I had to give my ID and was told to take a seat. I had been told to wear what I will wear on my head for the radiation treatments. I found that odd, but learned it had to do with positioning on the table. At this point I was literally bald. All my hair had come out during the chemo, and I wore my head wrapped in a scarf with a thin skullcap underneath to hold the scarf in place.

In the waiting room there were many ladies also waiting for radiation. In the Middle East at some facilities there are separate waiting rooms for women and men. The men's waiting room was down the hall. I walked into the women's waiting room and greeted everyone with a standard "salam alaykum" (peace be unto you/ hello); to which some whispered "walaikum salam" (and peace be unto you/hello). I took my seat and imagined each person's story as I am sure they were trying to figure out mine.

Ronnie's Words of Wisdom

I was taking Arabic lessons at the time. As I listened to the ladies in the waiting room chat, I could understand that some women only had a few more sessions to go and some were just getting started. Some looked tired, like me, and some looked very weak and exhausted. I also tried to muster up energy to "appear" to be feeling well so that I would feel better and NOT succumb to "looking like I had cancer." I wanted to project some positivity into the room. When you can, be the light for others. It will brighten your day too.

That first visit for radiation was very long. The technician, Talal, had to place small tattoo dots on my chest area (between my breasts) and under my arms and take various kinds of measurements for lining up the site for radiation. After this appointment for the following treatment sessions, these dots would be lined up with the lasers in the radiation room to ensure the correct spot was receiving the radiation. Wearing a head wrap that was bulky or large in the treatment room would mean that the technicians may not have been able to place me in the correctly aligned position for the treatment. There was a method to their madness.

As I was being aligned and tatted again, Talal was calling out numbers to his assistant in another room and making adjustments, as I lay on the table with my right breast exposed. He used some lasers to line up the breast. I also found out that the measurements from the MRI would be included to help with alignment. The process was all very regimented and sequenced. Talal worked efficiently to make sure that the right spot would be marked for radiation. He commented to me that this session would be the longest and that my subsequent sessions would be shorter. The whole procedure was about an hour, and I was tired.

I had timed how long it took me to get to the hospital from my home: forty-five minutes to the hospital and fifty minutes back. I was very doubtful as to whether I could do the drive every day for fifteen radiation treatments: drive, park, walk to the hospital, get the treatment, walk back and then drive home before my afternoon sessions began online. I did not think *The Beast* would allow that level of strength in me.

Knowing the procedure and having the information, I remember thinking to myself... "Self, I said, if you have to drive to the university for the treatment, park, walk to the building, have the treatment, walk back to the car and then drive home, you will be exhausted and may not have the energy for the afternoon clients." I had to think of another way to get the fifteen daily radiation treatments. Taking an Uber was out of the question. Remember, this was still during the pandemic, and I did not want to put myself at risk for COVID. Getting into an Uber and being exposed to COVID with my compromised immune system was not an option. Nor could I ask a friend to drive me, as I did not know who/where they had been to expose me to COVID. I had to find an alternative.

I decided that I needed help, so I asked Amina, the wife of my sponsor. She was in charge of the drivers of the cars of her household. I called her and told her about my dilemma with time and fatigue. Before I was finished, she had offered me a driver, Mr.

Mahmoud, for transportation to and from the university hospital for the radiation treatment for as long as I needed. Mr. Mahmoud had been vaccinated and was adhering to the COVID protocols, which were strict. Thank God! It eased my mind to know that I did not have to be attentive during the ride but could rest and relax instead.

I was so grateful that Amina had agreed to lend me one of her drivers for my radiation appointments. Just knowing that I did not have to make that drive in heavy traffic to and from the site helped me to get a little extra rest each way. If the drive was forty-five minutes; that was a good refreshing nap that I could use to quell *The Beast.* I was truly blessed to have the use of Mr. Mahmoud for my transportation.

THE FIRST RADIATION SESSION

The day had finally come for the first real radiation session. The appointment was for 10:00 a.m. The drive was a little dicey for that first session. Lots of stopping and starting and trying to get into correct lanes for turning. I laid my head back on the headrest of the seven-seater van as the driver navigated the roadway like a race car driver; steady and sure when he got the right of way. I arrived at the hospital in about thirty-five minutes—record time one could say. There was a semicircular drive that patients could be dropped off and Mr. Mahmoud let me out. I informed him that when I was finished, I would message him and meet him in the same place for the pick-up.

I tried to remember where the radiation room was. Chemo brain made my memory for recalling where to go foggy. I knew I needed to show my paperwork to gain entry to elevators that would take me downstairs to the area. The guard motioned me through after checking that I had an appointment at 10:00. Once I got off the elevator there was some signage that looked familiar, and I followed the directions. I arrived at the front desk and checked in and went to the waiting room. After about fifteen minutes, I was called back to the radiation room.

The radiation room was different from where I was measured and tatted. Extremely large doors could be seen on the left side of the room which led to the radiation room. The big doors seemed to lock with a seal when closed. I was met by two lovely female technicians. They were lively and fun and introduced themselves. Hanan was Middle Eastern who had lived in the US in California and had returned home to work, and Margaret was Canadian who had been in the Middle East for quite some time. The way they moved in sync and communicated with one another you could tell a few things about them: 1. They enjoyed their job; 2. They liked, respected and trusted each other, and 3. They liked to have fun while they worked. That was a perfect combination for me and made me feel comfortable. I had been blessed with another good patient-client relationship.

After introductions, I was asked to remove my top and my camisole and use the sheet for cover and come out of the dressing room and sit on the table and wait for instructions. The room was not terribly big, but the machine was huge and shaped weirdly. It had arms and wings that rotated about to deliver the radiation in the designated spot. The table was over size and long enough for me. As I got on the table and reclined, I could see lasers on the walls. The technicians later explained that this first session may take some time as they were rechecking the alignment, making more markings and being certain that the radiation was being delivered to the correct spot. They too called out numbers from the right and left sides of the table. One would say, "I have 96.5;" the other would say, "Wait a minute, I have to move it there, yep, got it 96.5." This went on for about fifteen minutes until they had me aligned properly to irradiate the area in my right breast of any remaining cancer cells that may have eluded the chemo and surgery. They added new markings on my right and left sides, just under my arm pits.

Radiation was about to begin. They told me to be very still, as I heard a humming sound come from the machine. The dose of radiation was being delivered. I tried to count how long it took, but I lost count after three minutes. Soon after that, maybe four minutes later, they said I was done and could get dressed. They let me know the next session would be fast as there was no need to get the measurements again, merely get lined up and deliver the radiation. THAT process was easy in comparison to the chemo. As I was getting dressed, I said a little prayer of thanks for the smooth procedure. I bid the technicians goodbye and told them I would see them tomorrow. I tried to send a message to Mr. Mahmoud, but the walls were so thick in that area that messages could not be received or sent. I waited until I got up to the ground floor and pushed the send message. As I walked out into the lobby, I saw people who were so ill and frail, some walking, some in wheelchairs being helped by family members or family helpers, I counted my blessings that I was still able to walk in and out of the hospital with no assistance and that I had a driver to get me back home safely.

Ronnie's Words of Wisdom

As I left the radiation area, I was counting my blessings. I did not feel tired. The process was not invasive. I just had to stay still on the table.

Radiation was the easy part of this protocol. I was feeling so fortunate to have gotten to this point with my complete clinical response to the chemo, a successful lumpectomy with no lymph nodes involved and most importantly, still working and moving forward each day, even though some days were hard. All in all, I was persevering in this journey. Remember, it is important to do a check in from time to time with yourself and recall just what you have gone through and survey where you are to gain appreciation for your accomplishments. Be thankful for being able to keep on keeping on in your journey—you are phenomenal!

The drive home was good. I remember thinking that I was so grateful I did not have to drive back to my flat. The traffic had picked up and it took about forty-five minutes to get back. At one point the traffic was so backed up that Mr. Mahmoud took another route to avoid the stopped traffic. I was watching and making note of the route so that I could use it if I were ever out and about and needed to get around a traffic jam.

Back at home, I had time for a nap before my afternoon sessions for speech therapy began. I quickly fell asleep and slept well.

ANOTHER BUMP IN THE ROAD

I woke up and got prepped for my afternoon sessions. This schedule went on for about nine treatment sessions. Then, the radiation machine broke. I got a call the day before one of my treatments from one of the technicians that the machine was broken and that they were waiting on a part. I asked if the break would be detrimental to my treatment, the technician assured me that it would not be harmful. I relished the days of not going for radiation and focused on getting stronger and eating healthy.

The break from radiation was about one week. I got a call on a Saturday night that I could come and resume my radiation treatments. I would stick to the same schedule that I had before. The radiation session ran like a well-oiled machine. Check in, wait, go back, remove shirt and camisole, get on table, get positioned and aligned, get radiation, get off table, put on camisole and shirt and call driver, drive home, nap, do afternoon sessions.

From 3 March 2021 until 28 March 2021, I had fifteen rounds of radiation. It was not painful or intrusive. It was the easiest part of my overall treatment. Just like on my last chemo session, on the day of my last radiation treatment, I brought Hanan, Margaret and Talal (who had measured me) a delicious date loaf from *Sucré Salé*. They were appreciative. For the ladies at the front desk and in the waiting room, I brought ma'amoul (date cookies) for them to enjoy. I was so happy to close that chapter of my treatment.

A few weeks later, I am coming out of the shower, and I notice there is a brown square/rectangle on my right breast—the spot where the radiation was given. I had only noticed a mild discoloration a few weeks prior, but this was a squarish rectangle on my right breast. I Googled to find out that would be a typical reaction from the radiation at the site of the treatment and it would fade in a few weeks, and it did. I took a deep breath, thanked God, and stepped into another day.

CHAPTER FOURTEEN

The Last Piece of the Puzzle

LITTLE DID I know the entire process of chemotherapy would be so long and intricate. From the extensive testing prior to actually getting started with treatment, then receiving the chemo and finally the testing after the chemo. The system of checks and balances left no stones unturned. I felt like I was in good hands—thank God!

Approximately two weeks after my final radiation treatment, I was scheduled for a Bone Mineral Density test (BMD). This was done as a baseline measurement of the density of my bones after exposure to chemotherapy. The BMD test looks at how dense (thick) my bones are and takes a measurement. It would also measure how much calcium and other types of minerals are in any area of my bones. One of the side effects of the chemo drugs that I took was osteopenia (aka brittle bones). The BMD would help the Oncologist and cancer team detect any osteopenia (loss of bone mineral density) or osteoporosis (bone break down) and predict my risk for bone fractures. This in turn would be tied directly to my calcium intake. I was already taking calcium supplements and getting Denosumab injections every six months as a prophylactic.

As was standard procedure, I drove myself to the hospital. The test was non-invasive and did not have to remove my clothes. I had never had a BMD done. My Momma had talked about hers and that she had been sore/stiff afterwards. I mentally prepped myself for something uncomfortable but was grateful it was anything but!

I entered the hospital Imaging waiting room as I had done on so many other occasions and waited for my number to be called. During COVID the hospital waiting rooms were always crowded. They had the seats blocked off so that every other seat was open; it was a form of social distancing. I always tried to arrive early and find a seat in the corner so I would be seated beside only one person. The wait was not long at all. When they called my name, I went back with the technician. I was given a liquid concoction to drink called radionuclide or tracer. I was not expecting that. It tasted chalky and thick, but I got through it in a few sips. Afterwards, I was told I had to go home and come back in two and a half hours for the scan. I was thanking God that I had a gap in my schedule that allowed this accommodation.

I drove back home, which was about five kilometers or a little over three miles like I was instructed to do. The way I had to drive home was convoluted and would take about twelve minutes. When I got home, I organized some files and of course, I Googled the tracer and effects of the drink. The tracer collects within the bone tissue at spots that may be abnormal physically or chemically. The tracer sends out a type of gamma radiation that is harmless. It's like when you see pictures of skeletons with black outlines. The only precaution mentioned was that I had to be certain I drank plenty of water afterwards to flush the tracer from my system.

Soon it was time to return to the hospital Imaging area. I drove back and was admitted straight to the scan area.

The Technician met me and asked me to remove my shoes. She asked if I had anything with buttons or zippers and I did not, as I had read that those types of clothing items were not allowed in the testing. I hopped up on the table. She told me to be very still during the procedure, as good images of the bones were needed for analysis of the density.

The machine was akin to a giant scanner. It had a large C-shaped arm that extended over the table. It was able to slide up and down the sides of the table taking images of my bones. It was pain free and you guessed it- I went to sleep during the procedure. I was still experiencing chemo related fatigue and anytime my body was not in motion, it was a sign to relax and nap. I could hear the faint hum of the scanner as it lulled me into relaxation and a short nap. At the beginning of the test, I had looked at the technician's desk and monitor to see if I could see what she was seeing but I could not. I had to wait until the test was completed. I asked if I could see what she was looking at. She said she was not supposed to show or make any interpretations, but she allowed me to peek.

The scan of my bones looked like something from a Halloween horror movie. A long skeletal image was on one screen, on another was a scan of my femur bones. Some of the images were zoomed in so that the density of the bones could be seen. The bone density looked like a honeycomb pattern. The technician said that the images would be read and analyzed, and a report would be generated in two days. The calculated numbers from the scan would be taken and stored for later analysis and comparison. At some point the procedure could be repeated if needed and the numbers compared for analysis to determine changes in my bone mass density after a sequence of treatments. This is a pretty good system of checks and balances for my health! The results would be available in two days. I would have to wait patiently.

I never really thought about how strong my bones are. I know they support me and that from time to time I get a little ache in a joint. I never focused on my bones, until now when I could find out I had brittle bones, yet another thing on top of the cancer. I had to just wait and see, When the results were available, I used a reference guide to help me understand the numbers. It was important to know and understand the information about MY body.

Having doses of chemo for breast cancer, as well as other types of cancer can significantly decrease your calcium. My calcium levels were affected and thus the Denosumab addition to my protocol. I also was taking a calcium supplement (800mg of calcium; 300mg magnesium; 10mg zinc and 5 micrograms of vitamin D) during and after the chemo to keep my calcium levels stable.

The numbers were calculated using T-scores and Z-scores. These T-scores compared my bone mass to that of a healthy young adult. The "T" represents the number of standard deviations (variation of the average) or units of measurement my score is above or below the average bone density of a young healthy adult. Scores were calculated for my spine, left and right femoral neck (hip joint), as well as my left and right femur. An estimated ten-year risk would be calculated based on those numbers to indicate my risk for fractures, in particular hip fractures All of my T scores were -1.3 or less. These scores indicated that I had low bone mass; although not low enough to be diagnosed as osteoporosis, but rather *osteopenia*.

My Z-scores were -1.7 or less. The Z-scores compared my bone density to the average values for a person of my same age and gender. The scores fell within the range of having low bone mass for my expected age. The T and Z scores would be used in calculating the *Trabecular Bone Score* (**TBS**). This score represents the internal structure of the bones at a microscopic level. These were the honeycomb images of my bones that I saw when the technician allowed me to look at the monitor. Another calculation done was something called a Fracture Risk Assessment Tool (FRAX). A FRAX is a risk calculator that calculates your chances of having different types of fractures. My TBS was 4.3 % for major osteoporotic fracture and .4% for hip fracture. That's relatively low for a person of my age at the time (62 years old). I interpreted this to mean my bones had not significantly been impacted by the chemo or radiation. My bone density would and will always be followed because of my exposure to the chemo and immunotherapy after the chemo and radiation. My Oncologist and the Cancer Counselor were glad I was continuing my daily workouts with weight bearing exercises to strengthen my bones and my body and taking my calcium supplements. This too I was committed to overcoming.

CHAPTER FIFTEEN

This Feels Very Familiar

I T MIGHT FEEL like I have been rattling off an endless list of procedures, treatments, and tests up until this point but there's more. In fact, the protocol for the next steps requires a second round of testing. These tests are done at the end of six months after the the chemo, surgery and radiation. Since I was familiar with the process, I knew how to get approval prior to the procedures, and I knew the time they would take so that I could incorporate the appointments into my schedule. I scheduled the ultrasound and mammogram on the same day and then two days later, I scheduled the MRI and CT scan.

The ultrasound was first. The sonographer did my left breast first. In the initial ultrasound and in the one right after the chemo, the left breast was done rather quickly. This time it was not so fast.

Remember that a mass was seen in the last ultrasound and MRI that was of little or no concern, as it had not taken on contrast in the MRI and was not cancerous. Now, in the new ultrasound, the mass was once again detected, and the sonographer was trying to get a good view of it for the Radiologist. I understood and was praying everything would be ok.

Ronnie's Words of Wisdom

After being diagnosed with breast cancer, any lump, bump, funny feeling, twinge, or sharp pain automatically took me to the question: "Is that related to my cancer?" I was in hyper awareness mode and always trying to tune into what my body was telling me. Little did I know this would be my new way of life until well after all my procedures were completed. I would be living as a breast cancer survivor in remission when a five-year period was over without an incidence of cancer. Only then could I be considered cured. I longed for THAT day.

The sonographer finally got a satisfactory image of the left breast and moved on to my right breast. This time, the right breast ultrasound was fast, as the mass had been destroyed by the chemo and was nowhere to be found—thank God. My concern and attention NOW was for the **left** breast.

Dr. Noura, my Radiologist, entered the room. She was dressed sharply in pumps and a Versace dress and her crisp white lab coat. We had a pleasant greeting. She congratulated me on my complete clinical response to the chemo for the right breast. Dr. Noura then began to talk about my left breast, however, she prefaced it by saying in a very emphatic way that she did not think the mass that was seen in my left breast was malignant, as it did not have the consistency, but it warranted a biopsy. I knew the procedure for the biopsy. I got approval and went to another room for the procedure to begin.

Dr. Noura gave me the anesthesia to numb my left breast and waited a few minutes until I felt nothing. She then took the long probe and inserted it into my breast at about the two o'clock position and took the sample. She placed the sample in a specimen jar. I think Dr. Noura read the worry on my face after she took the sample. She once again told me not to worry about this one, as she said it was different from the other specimen. I believed her, but still had a bit of doubt to creep into my thoughts. I resorted to prayer that God's will be done. Again, I would have to wait two days for the results to come in. I did not share that I had another biopsy with My Tribe. Cannot tell you why, except maybe, I did not want them to worry for no reason, as Dr. Noura was pretty certain, the mass was benign and just a fibroadenoma. I just prayed and waited for the results.

The mammogram was fast and easy. The technician placed colorful little pieces of radiopaque marker tape on my nipples and on the lumpectomy scar so that the sites would be seen and discerned on the film of the mammogram. The skin markers would not hide any breast tissue, but merely mark the areas for reading the film adequately. After getting my body into the proper position and having the breasts placed and pressed onto the tray, the mammogram was quick. First the left breast, then the right—easy peasy!

Ronnie's Words of Wisdom

I was accustomed to the procedures for the
ultrasound and mammogram, as I had them
done a few times now. I think I gained a level of
comfort for having the tests done just as you do
with being familiar with something. It was a no
worry—it has to be done attitude. I have always
been comfortable about my body with doctors but
during my journey there was this feeling of "tell
me what you need to see, and I will show you."
For the doctors to have complete access to what
they needed to see and do, I needed to have some
confidence in showing them. This feeling just came
with the territory of dealing with a breast cancer
diagnosis. I had placed my breasts into the hands
(literally) of the medical team for them to do as
they needed to get me well. You'll get used to it all,
I promise.

A few days later, I had the MRI and the CT repeated—nothing
new about the procedures. I was more than grateful for having
done the procedures before and knowing what to expect. In the
MRI tunnel, I did not have the nausea I had the first time. I had
learned to close my eyes upon entry and just relax. I was able to get
myself so relaxed that I fell asleep. I had to have the contrast for this
MRI too, so two times into the machine. Both times I just slept.

Both rounds of the CT (with and without contrast) were
uneventful, and it did not seem to take as long, as the first one. It
was somewhat interesting, as I recall, how my mind raced during

the first time I had a procedure that I was not familiar with. Now, I had a relaxed approach to it, and it went rather smoothly.

THE WAITING GAME

Waiting for the results was something I had become accustomed to, but with this round of tests, my mind was more on my CRF and neuropathy, and maneuvering through each. Before I knew it, the results were back—all clear: biopsy—revealed a fibroadenoma of the left breast; MRI—no signs of any cancer anywhere in my body; CT—all clear. I fell on my knees for a prayer of gratitude after reading the reports in the app on my phone. I was appreciative of the level of care I received and would continue to receive in this journey. Now I could focus on getting my energy back and dealing with my foot and hand neuropathy. It would be weeks until I shared the facts that I had another biopsy with My Tribe. It was something that I needed to do, to protect them from worrying. That is okay.

Ronnie's Words of Wisdom

I am not going to tell you that I did not worry about the results of this biopsy. I did. What concerned me was there was a chance that I would have to do an encore performance of my cancer journey. I asked myself if was up for the task. I finally told myself that if indeed I had to go through chemo, surgery, etc., that I would do it all again and document just as I had done this time. I assured myself that together God, My Tribe and I would find a way to do it all again. I only knew how to pray, persevere and stay positive in this journey. As I said before, you find the sheer will to keep moving forward and just keep going.

THE ONE-YEAR MILESTONE

Now that the protocol after all the testing was done, I had to keep taking the Denosumab injections every six months. I also had to have a hormone medication to keep my hormones and proteins at bay. I will take letrozole (Femara) daily for five years to block the production of estrogen so that no stimulation of my hormone receptors would occur to make cancer cells. My time frame for testing would now be yearly ultrasounds and mammograms only. This was a feat in and of itself. I remember my Oncologist talking about this moment of long-term care, but it seemed so far off—I had made it to this milestone in my treatment.

CHAPTER SIXTEEN

My Letter to You

DEAR FRIENDS ON a Cancer Journey,

I am healthy today and forever changed.

As I draw upon the completion of my book, I still find it utterly fascinating that I am now considered a *cancer survivor*. It's even recondite for me to write those two words **cancer** and **survivor**. I am grateful, blessed, fortunate, and most of all overjoyed that I have been able to share my story with you.

With you reading through my journey, this has bonded us. You have gained insights into my medical, mental, physical, emotional, spiritual and philosophical well-being. It is my hope that you have gleaned information to share and use accordingly on your journey or with someone you love. My sole purpose in writing this book was to show how I managed life during my cancer journey and to inspire you to do the same. I am forever changed by my cancer diagnosis.

One year passed so quickly. Now, it has been almost three (two years and nine months exactly) since my first round of chemotherapy during a pandemic in a foreign country. That fact is still hard for me to fathom and grasp. Almost three years ago my life changed with a diagnosis of Intraductal Carcinoma. I demonstrated endurance and persistence in my journey. God is good, all the time. All the time, God is good.

My journey was the most strenuous thing I have ever done. However, it was not so hard that I ever wanted to surrender to this dreaded disease. That was not a part of who I had been rehearsing to be all my life. "Fight" was all I knew, and that is what I did with the help of my prayers to God, My Tribe, and an amazing medical team.

If I described how I am doing now it would be "exceptionally well." I say "exceptionally well" because going through this journey in the Middle East during a pandemic is an exception to the rule. My cancer journey was anything but typical. Having cancer is out of the ordinary. If you have to deal with cancer, you are an exception to that rule; and therefore, your status of being is "exceptionally well!"

I repeat, I am blessed to have had a magnificent medical team who listened to my concerns and guided me during my journey. I cannot stress how important it is for you to get your annual mammograms and self-advocate to gain a level of knowledge about your cancer. It is imperative you fully take part in your treatment— it really is all about you; why not invest in yourself?

Medically, I will be on my five-year regime of drugs to prevent my cancer from recurring. I am taking Femara (aka letrozole), calcium and supplements, Omega 3, Denosumab (injection; every six months), and Amlor for hypertension. I am extremely vigilant in taking my meds. I need to keep the proteins from being made by my body that the cancer likes to dine on. My meds are located in a convenient and visible place in my bedroom to ensure I take them each morning.

Because of my cancer journey, I am so much more aware how my body feels. I have always taken pride in listening to my body, a trait I got from my Momma. Nowadays, when I have a twinge, ache or just feel uneasy about something, I am trying to determine the root cause and act accordingly. This skill was so important during my journey, as I was tuned into how tired my body was. However, I knew I needed to keep moving so my muscles did not tighten or cease up. This mindset of pushing myself I believe stems from years of seeing my parents persevere and then years of athletic training, pushing to get that last rep in or that surge you had to have to make a timed run quota. As I said earlier, I have been rehearsing for this performance all my life and I am so grateful I was able to connect it with my journey.

From a physical perspective, I am moving and doing many of things that I did pre-cancer. As you know, during my cancer journey, I continued my daily workouts and weightlifting to ensure I had maintained my stamina to drive myself to my treatments/appointments. I will forever deeply believe that keeping this regime was instrumental in my overall physical stability to fight my cancer. I moved about **each and every day**; I was not sedentary. I could not afford to be, as I needed to be ambulatory to get myself to and from my appointments.

Keep moving every day, you will be glad you did when it is all said and done. Remember: Move It or Lose It!

My tell-tale signs of cancer will remain for a while, so I have read. I am not talking about the scars—they will be my gentle reminders that I was in a battle for my life; and won! I am referring to the neuropathy and the cancer related fatigue that continues to overtake my body months post cancer. They batter my body each and every day; and each and every day I meet the challenge and get through it. I continue to golf almost every weekend and walk twenty minutes or more each day. Some days, I golf and walk easily, some days, I am more aware of where my feet are and how to position them for a solid gait.

I want you to be in the moment and develop the fortitude to get through that moment and then go to the next. Keep doing what you do, and the day will have gone by without you even realizing you have conquered another day. This has worked for me. It is my hope that you too can adopt this mentality for being in the moment and moving forward.

From a professional perspective, I continue to see my clients. Some are online and some are face to face. I did not cancel many sessions during my bout with cancer. I truly believe that having a workload and needing to show up every day was my personal motivation. This obligation helped me to keep my cancer in clear focus. I knew I had to provide a service to others and that in turn was rewarding for me.

As I have said earlier, try to keep to some type of daily routine. It will give you purpose and not allow you time to dwell on your cancer. Channel that energy into positive thoughts about getting well and how your life will be changed after this experience.

Now for the emotional perspective. You will undergo a physical healing as well as a soulful healing. This is probably the most dramatically changed part of me. I have always been an intellectual thinker in times of crisis; my emotions are on the back burner until the crisis is solved and under control. Now, the emotional/soulful aspect is allowing me to go to a deep level of feeling commonly referred to in the cancer world as *benefit finding*. I am finding that I have made a dynamic paradigm shift in my overall thinking and perception from an emotional standpoint. I feel a great deal of intensity of any emotion now whether it be happiness, sadness, fear, disgust, anger or surprise. All of my emotions are heightened with a deep sense of connection. At the same time, I am now able to put emotions in perspective and ask myself "Is it really worth the (emotion) at the time?" I seem to always have this caveat in my thinking that helps to quell any overreaction. Having cancer has allowed me to stop and ask, "In the grand scheme, is this enough of a difference to make a difference?" My response to that question is now typically... "nahhhh, it's just not that serious!" As the old cliché goes "Life is too short." Having faced a life changing challenge, I will no longer waste time on trivial things.

My Friends, it goes without saying that having cancer **will** change you. I have embraced my change. You should too. It is now a fabric of my being I am proud of. I welcome, with confidence, the continued changes I am sure to have along the way in all areas of my being. That is my hope for you as well.

I know that I had this cancer experience for a reason or reasons. I know for sure one reason was so that I could inspire and encourage you to keep up the fight and find that inspiration by reading my book. I am absolutely positive that other reasons will be revealed to me when the times are right, and I am ready.

Finally, if you are in your cancer journey, I have a prayer for you: I pray that your medical, mental, physical, spiritual, philosophical and emotional health will be exceptional and ongoing. I pray that reading about my journey has helped you gain some awareness and strength for your journey. It is also my prayer that if you are a caregiver or family member reading this book that you have gained insights into what your loved one has/is experienced/ing. It will be important that you have a perspective to be there for them and provide whatever support is needed at any time. Showing up will be most appreciated in an immeasurable way by your loved one going through this battle.

Stay strong! Be aware, prayerful and insightful! Keep moving forward!

Let me know how things are going—please send me an email at info@ronnielaughlin.com.

May you always remember that this journey is all about **YOU!**

—Love,

Ronnie

Acknowledgements

When I was first diagnosed with breast cancer during the 2020 pandemic, I knew that what I was about to go through was not going to be any run of the mill experience. I was not fully aware of what or how the pandemic would impact my treatment, but I knew that I would need to stay as healthy as possible. When I knew that my treatment plan included chemotherapy, I knew that as a consequence, my immune system would eventually be comprised. I would need to be extremely cautious with who I interacted with. I began to think that I would need to keep track of what was happening to me, as I remembered my friends who had cancer who mentioned "chemo brain" and not remembering things. I had been journaling all along just to keep track of my life, now I would journal with purpose and for later reference. My journaling would also be a link to acknowledging the people who impacted my life during my journey.

I would be remiss if I began without mentioning My Heavenly Father, Son, Holy Spirit and Mary to whom I prayed each day. As a praying Catholic, I had my litany of prayers from having His will be done to Mary also intervening. I prayed and hoped that I would get another day. I always did and for that, I am more than thankful. It is my belief that God allowed me to have this journey to write about it, to publish a book, and to help others. It was through His grace and mercy that I am writing this book now.

Because I chose to tell a small subset of people about my breast cancer diagnosis, there was a small circle of people that provided support and encouragement for me. I will be ever so appreciative of that love and support.

When I told My Tribe, about my diagnosis and that I would later write a book, they all said, "That's a great idea" and encouraged me. For that support I am filled with gratitude and feel the need to thank them and so many others who made this book possible. I have to go on record that I have the most supportive family and circle of friends. They were the source of my internal motivation to keep moving forward.

I only told my Sister, Edwina Brown, in my family. Edwina was one of my biggest cheerleaders. She had a knack for sending quips to uplift me and when we chatted always telling me to keep on going with her "Sistah Girl" comments. She gave me insightful hints about how to manage my health; having been through similar circumstances as our Mother's Caregiver. Thanks for your daily prayers, messages and encouragement.

Now to My Tribe: Angie Martin, Angela Lott-Bower, Ben Bower, and Jennifer Reeves. My heart is full of love and appreciation for each and every one of you.

Angie, you kept me prayed up. Your check-ins and ultimatums if you did not hear from me after a couple of days always made me smile; I knew you cared about me and loved me. You gave me room to be "Ronnie" and you understood the assignment. I am so happy that Dr. Freda Wilson had us meet. You really are my Sister from another Mother!

Angela, you were my sounding board for all the medical stuff I faced. When you volunteered to come and be with me for my surgery I breathed a sigh of relief, for I knew that your Registered Nursing eyes would be all over me during my hospital stay and after—you made me feel safe and for that I am grateful. Who knew that we would meet seven thousand miles from Greensboro, NC where we grew up a few miles from one another? You were my other Sister from another Mother.

Ben, your prayers and encouragement were felt whenever we Face Timed. Your words and witty comments were a welcome relief during my journey. My heart smiled when we chatted. I am grateful that I had you as one of my Prayer Warriors.

Jen, our weekly chats kept me looking forward to hearing from you and seeing Niblets's ears perk up when he heard my voice. Our chats always brightened my day, as we reminisced about our shopping antics of the past. Your gifts of the camisoles were a blessing when I had my horrible rash all over my upper body and could not wear a bra. The camisoles were a godsend, and I am thankful that you shared your Amazon finds with me.

I had another group of friends that I communicated with during and after my journey. They too were in the small subset. Pamela Lesmond, Sage Park, Cathy Zachary, Dr. Sandra-Eric Braham, Colette Glover-Hannah and Dr. Monica Cherry.

Pam, you were on this journey well before me and we always compared notes. You guided me through some low energy days and kept me thinking about getting well. As my hairdresser, I had trusted you from years ago and you were the one who guided me when it was time to shave my head. You asked me several times "Girl, you sure you ready?" and you gave me some good pointers in how to get a good shave. I was thankful to have you in my circle for your insights, understanding and experienced guidance.

Sage, we chatted nearly everyday during my journey and you always asked how I was and if I needed anything. Your lovely gesture of leaving the beautiful purple orchid at my flat for me when

I returned from surgery warmed my heart. I thank you for your willingness to help in any way possible.

Cathy, you were another one of my Prayer Warriors that I am grateful for. Our weekly chats always led us back to some funny incidents that we have shared over the years. I thank you for your ability to get me to laugh during my journey and I appreciate our long friendship.

Dr. Sandra-Eric Braham, thanks for your insights and direction when I decided to write this book. Seeing your success was encouraging. I thank you for your willingness to share your tricks of the trade about how your book, *An Angel for Detroit*, was published. You supported all my questions about the publishing process. You were an inspiration and I thank you.

Colette Glover-Hannah, you were so matter of fact in your support when I shared about my journey and that I wanted to write a book. You told me that I could write a book. Your even keel approach to life was a godsend. As an author of, *MomPrenure; Managing Partnerships, Parenthood and Presentations*, you gave me suggestions tips and ideas to safely negotiate the publishing waters. You were a great golf partner too when I came home. Our long chats solving the world's problems were a blessing. Your never-ending drive and determination to be more and better was always a hashtag goal of mine. I thank you for being the living example of how to have it all.

Dr. Cherry, thank you for your adept clinical skills for allowing me to check-in mentally with you to stay on the right path and manage my feelings about my cancer and writing/editing and all that comes with writing a book. Your guided questions and thought-provoking comments always gave me room for pause. I am grateful that we connected. Your skills are invaluable in keeping me grounded, focused and handling my life in the best way possible for me.

WRITING A BOOK TAKES A VILLAGE

Francesca, we only had one meeting. You helped me lay the groundwork for my book. You had pre-read some chapters and immediately told me that readers would want to know where I came from, what made me, me. I knew that your keen sense of knowing what the readers wanted was valuable. I am filled with gratitude that we met and that you set me on the right path for my book. Thanks for your direction.

Maureen Petrosky, I was grateful you came on board with your book writing and publishing experience. You jumped right in and gave some good directions on my content. Your first email to me was uplifting when you commented about my writing style. I loved how you set up your boundaries and laid out your style. I am a rule follower and enjoyed the guides. In the first edits, you emailed and prepared me for the edits by letting me know that even though there was a great deal of "red" (edits), all the information was there; just moved to a new location. You put me at ease about the editing process. You always had valid responses to my questions and allowed me to have my freedom to say things in a certain way. I am indebted to you for your exceptional editing skills and for seeing this book to fruition.

Rick Benitez Photography thanks for your efforts with my photos. Your directions during the photo shoot made it easy and fun.

Jerry Brunson at Brunson Photography your willingness to do a photo shoot spur of the moment for me yielded great photos. Thanks. Your effort will always be much appreciated.

Profound thanks to Heidi Jensen for introducing me to Scott Spiewak of Franklin Green Publishing. Heidi, your quick thinking and creative insights were a godsend. Scott your eagerness to take on my project was most appreciated. Thanks also to Kent Jensen for your keen eye for details for the cover and typesetting; you worked a miracle with having the pages stand out. Team Franklin Green Publishing, you are exceptional and made completing my book a smooth task.

Nora Lynn Finch, thank you for writing my foreword. When I contacted you to ask if you would write the foreword, you did not hesitate or shy away from the task—that was never your style! I am grateful for you Nora Lynn in so many ways. I knew that I was in good hands when I signed to play basketball for you at Peace College in 1976. During my college career at Peace and North Carolina State University your care, guidance and tutelage enhanced my social, emotional, spiritual and physical well-being to provide a solid foundation for navigating the world. I am forever grateful to you for that. I have cherished our friendship over the years and I am extremely thankful to have you in my life. Thank you for writing such a touching and adept foreword for my book.

I cannot go any further without acknowledging my sponsor, Hamza and his wife, Amina who employed me in the Middle East and provided me with a good insurance plan that allowed me to have excellent medical care during my journey. They were willing to accommodate me in any way through my journey; I will be forever grateful for the immeasurable generosity. Having access to your driver for my radiation treatments was a godsend. Thank you for making this journey "doable" while I still worked.

I am so appreciative of the level of medical care I received in the Middle East. All of my doctors were amazing. They all worked together as a very cohesive team to provide some very top-tier treatment with a positive outcome for me. I am thankful that all my medical team valued my input and saw me as a person. They made me feel like I had their attention in all matters. My medical team was amazing. Thank you for your exceptional standard of care.

The Nurses in Oncology were some of the best. I thank you for your cheerfulness, gentleness and ability to answer my many questions during my chemo process. You were the most kind and compassionate Nurses I have ever been around. Thanks for your stellar skills and service.

I have to acknowledge the Insurance Claims Agents who navigated my approvals for my services. Their savviness and expertise were highly appreciated.

I do not want to do a Snoop Dogg maneuver here, but I do want to acknowledge myself for staying in the moment during my journey and having faith that I would get through this journey. I had to slow down and just reflect and focus on where I had been, who I had been associated with, what had been done, the manner in which it was done and then pray for the plan to come to fruition. Again, I am grateful for God's grace, mercy, guidance and strength in my journey. After all, this was an atypical journey that I had rehearsed for all my life.

Glossary of Terms

Adjuvant Therapy: A primary type of treatment that involves surgery first for the excision of the tumor, then radiation as prophylaxis (prevention).

Anesthesia (propofol): A drug used to induce sleep during surgery.

Angiogram: A way to view blood vessels for guidance during various procedures.

Benign: Non-cancerous.

BIRADS: Breast Imaging Reporting Data System. A system that categorizes breast images. The categories range from 0 (findings are unclear; more images are needed) to 6 (cancer was diagnosed using a biopsy).

Bone Scintigraphy: A bone scan is a specialized radiology procedure used to examine the various bones of the skeleton. It is done to identify areas of physical and chemical changes in bone. A bone scan may also be used to follow the progress of treatment of certain conditions.

BRCA: Breast Cancer gene test. It is used to determine the presence of BRCA 1 or BRCA 2 gene.

BRCA 1 Gene: Linked to triple negative breast cancer—a very aggressive and deadly form of breast cancer that can increase the risk of ovarian, pancreatic, gallbladder, bile duct and melanoma cancers. Usually inherited.

BRCA 2 Gene: Associated with cancer that are generally estrogen receptor positive.

Cancer-Related Fatigue (CRF): Extreme and long-lasting fatigue associated with chemotherapy. It is unlike fatigue from being tired; sleep does not help CRF.

CBC (complete blood count): Blood analysis done to determine blood cell count. CBC is monitored during chemo to ensure adequate white blood cell count.

Clip/Marker: A marker placed subcutaneously (under the skin) that helps the surgeon more easily find the site when surgery is warranted for breast cancer.

Contrast: Liquid material injected into the vein via an IV (intravenous) to help highlight any abnormal areas of breast tissue or any other abnormal tissue during an MRI (magnetic resonance image) or CT scan. The ingredient in the contrast is called gadolinium.

Core Needle Biopsy: A hollow needle that is used to remove pieces of breast tissue.

CT (computerized tomography) Scan: A scan typically done to diagnose tumors, investigate internal bleeding, or check for internal injuries or damage. The scan combines a series of x-ray images from different angles around the body. Computer processing is used to create cross sectional images or slices of the tissue they are focusing on. The CT scan gives more detailed information than a plain X-ray. The CT scan is considered an asset to the cancer profession for its detailed imaging.

Dexamethasone: Drug used during chemotherapy to help quell nausea and vomiting. It can also be used for other medical ailments such as allergies, asthma, and skin diseases.

Echocardiogram (ECHO): A graphic outline of the movement of the heart's valves and chambers through the use of a hand-held wand guided over the chest assessing the heart's anatomy and function.

Fibroadenoma: A solid, not fluid filled tumor caused by a deviation or change during normal development of breast tissue. The breast lobules become hyperplastic (over plastic). This change can be related to estrogen, progesterone, pregnancy and lactation.

Filgrastim: A drug that stimulates bone marrow to make new white blood cells that are measured via the white blood count (WBC).

Gait: Your walking strides.

Heparin: An anticoagulant (prevents blood clotting). It is used in the port-a-catheter to keep it open or patent between chemo treatments.

HER: Human Epidermal growth factor Receptor (a protein).

HER 2: A protein that promotes the growth of cancer cells.

Immunohistochemistry (IHC): A test used to determine cell type and organ of origin. The test can be performed on breast tissue samples that are suspected of being malignant (cancerous). The sample may be tested for HER2 receptors and/or hormone receptors.

In situ: Original place.

Intraductal Carcinoma: Aka, ductal carcinoma in situ (DCIS); cancer in its original place; it has not spread.

Intravenous: In the vein.

Keloids: Thick raised scar on skin.

Lesion: A tumor.

Mammogram: A visual representation of the breasts using various views to discern the structure/landscape of the breast and determine the tissue, density, identify masses and locate malignant and benign masses in the breast. Low-energy X-rays are used to examine the breast for diagnosis or screening or the location of a marker for future surgery.

Margins: Typical, a rim of tissue around the site anywhere from 1-2 millimeters in circumference.

Metastasized: Spread.

Methylene Blue Dye: A dye injected into sentinel nodes which has radioactive properties to detect cancer. The dye can be seen in urine after being flushed from body.

Mucositis: The inflammation of the mucosal (mouth) region.

Neoadjuvant Therapy: A type of chemotherapy approach that is used ahead of surgery to help shrink a cancerous tumor or even kill cancerous tissue that is not visible on imaging tests. When neoadjuvant therapy is used, doctors may also be looking at how the tumor responds to the drugs, and this can guide the treatment.

Neutropenia: Low white blood cell count.

Nystagmus: Rapid side-to-side uncontrolled eye movements.

Olanzapine: A drug used in chemotherapy treatment to quell nausea and vomiting.

Osteopenia: Brittle bones.

Palpate: To touch.

Patent: To keep open.

Pathogens: Germs.

Port-a-Catheter: A device that is inserted under the skin opposite the cancerous site that delivers chemotherapy drugs without harming veins in the patient. It is connected to the large vein that leads to the heart for distribution of the drugs throughout the body.

Positive Prognostic Indicators: Factors that contribute to good outcomes after treatment, e.g., healthy status, good diet, no history of illnesses.

Positive/Complete Clinical Response (P/CCR): Evidence that a tumor/lesion has been resolved (dissolved) after chemotherapy. The cancer is no longer detectable at the site.

Prophylactic: Just in case/preventative.

Prophylaxis: Prevention.

Sentinel Node: The first node located under the arm pit that a tumor will spread to. It is tested to determine if cancer is in other nodes in the lymph system.

Sonogram: Use of sound waves to see structures/organs.

Subcutaneous: Under the skin; a pocket made under the skin to insert a device.

Tumor Board: A group of hospital professionals consisting of Pathologists, Surgeons, Medical and Radiation Oncologists, Plastic Surgeons, Urologists, Gynecologists, Genetic counselor; and anyone else specific for the type of cancer of the patient in various areas of Oncology and Medicine. They typically meet weekly to discuss all cancer cases at a hospital and to determine the best possible cancer treatment and care plan for an individual patient, based on the most current research and best evidence-based practices.

Wire Localization: Use of a fine wire to mark the site of a tumor. It can guide the surgeon to ensure that they have the correct spot to remove the tissue or for the biopsy.

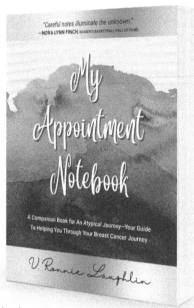

"Careful notes illuminate the unknown."
—NORA LYNN FINCH, WOMEN'S BASKETBALL HALL OF FAME

My
Appointment
Notebook

A Companion Book for An Atypical Journey—Your Guide
To Helping You Through Your Breast Cancer Journey

V. Ronnie Laughlin

VRL ©
RonnieLaughlin.com

My Appointment Notebook
V. Ronnie Laughlin

Are you or someone you love walking through breast cancer?

If so, *My Appointment Notebook* is for you. *My Appointment Notebook* is a comprehensive companion for all your appointment needs during your breast cancer journey. It provides the necessary support and organization to help you navigate through this difficult time by making your journey through cancer easier. It is a great resource full of gentle reminders, guidelines, and directions to help you ask the right questions and get the answers needed from your providers. All while keeping track of your appointments, tests, and medical procedures in one spot. You will not want to leave home without *My Appointment Notebook*—it is an essential tool to help you get through your breast cancer appointments.

My Appointment Notebook is Filled With:
- Impactful Guides
- Inspirational Quotes
- Insightful Encouragement
- Well-Structured and Organized Appointment Sheets—Located In One Place

To schedule an interview or speaking engagement please contact:
Heidi Jensen at heidifreshimpactpr@gmail.com

"When Life Kicks You, Let It Kick You Forward!"
-Kay Yow

10% of Proceeds Goes to
Kay Yow Cancer Fund.

Kay Yow Cancer Fund

4804 Page Creek Lane, Suite 118

Durham, NC 27703

Website: kayyow.com

Jenny Palmateer, CEO

"Your Attitude Determines Your Altitude."
-Kay Yow